7GOLDEN RULES of
ZEN
WISDOM

The revelations of truth that will heal
the negative conditioning of the mind.

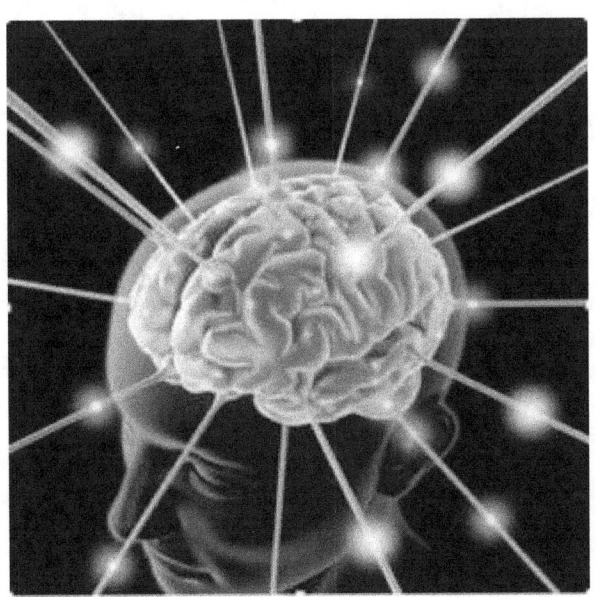

Publishers

Jay Kay®

Administrative office and sale center

HRBR Layout, Bangalore-560043

E-mail: info@authorjaykay.com • *Website:* www.authorjaykay.com

Edition: 2015

Printed at : Ar International, New Delhi

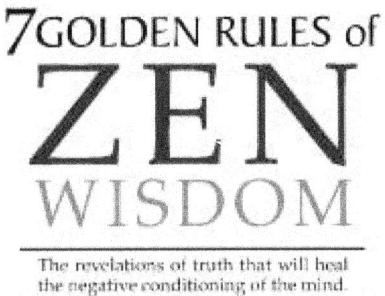

7GOLDEN RULES of
ZEN
WISDOM

The revelations of truth that will heal
the negative conditioning of the mind.

Jay Kay

(Author of Anna Heliott, A Lonely Survivor)

Publishers
Jay Kay®

Administrative office and sale centre
HRBR Layout, Bangalore-560043
E-mail: info@authorjaykay.com • *Website:* www.authorjaykay.com

© **Jay Kay,** Bangalore

Edition: 2015

Printed at: New Delhis

Preface

'7 Golden Rules of Zen Wisdom' describe the mind that has the ability to expand to the Super Consciousness. This compilation is based on a true story of transformation and research conducted in the US. You have a choice to expand mind to the Ultimate. The revelations of truth will heal your negative conditioning. This is an invitation to explore the 'SIXTH SENSE', The Mind, which is a hidden splendor in the abyss of the consciousness.

It deepened my awareness while I was reflecting my conditioning, about the mind, and the research took me beyond analyzing the human behavioral pattern, to the evolution of consciousness.

The transformation will start by realizing the fundamental values of truth, by analyzing the Sixth Sense. The sixth sense is lying dormant, without realizing the lineage to the supreme consciousness. This is a practical guide to self-healing and managing your mind to unleash its potential to succeed.

This book is an analysis of the past conditioning, and the human behavioral pattern to the revelations of inner consciousness. 'The 7 Golden Rules of Zen Wisdom' will help you transcend the conditioning, to uncover the truth. You will be able to achieve success by effectively managing the senses.

Dedication

To my beloved Guru, Enlightened Master,

Maharishi Vethathiri, who is an eternal love! The one who has helped many scientists in realization of truth.

Thank you! Without your support, I would have never achieved my dream.

Acknowledgements

I would like to thank my family, classmates, spiritual companion, friends, and leaders who've inspired me always and without whose help this book would never have been completed.

I would like to thank Dr. Madhavan (CEO, BIST, India), my friends, Sukumar Subramanian (CEO, VMG Entertainment, India), Chandrasekar Papudesu (Director, IBMUS) and Louis Victor Jayaraj (Sr. Director, Huawei India Technologies Ltd.) for their valuable feedback and suggestions to improve the manuscript.

Above all, thanks to my publishers, M/s Pustak Mahal in bringing life to my words!

Thank you for your patience and guidance.

Contents

Prologue 'Awareness Institute'

"Aloud announcement in the CNN auditorium filled with celebrities and hollywood actors."

Laura was flipping through the nominations card, and finally called out the name loudly. The CNN Humanitarian services AWARD for the year 2035 goes to Mr. Martin, founder of the Awareness Institute in the United States. Mr. Martin is a pioneer in helping thousands of young students become great leaders all over the world."

A three minutes video portraying Mr. Martin's achievements – Thousands of students all over the world, cheering him in the workshop presentations.

"May I request Mr. Martin to come on stage to receive the **2035-CNN AWARD** for the humanitarian services, by conducting thousands of workshops in East Africa to the United States. It has helped over a million viewers watching his programme through CNN broadcasts, podcasts and online meetings. These workshops have helped them get over addictions. Many have transformed themselves into leaders and top executives in every field."

I would like to introduce Mr. Martin who has been instrumental in helping students in every corner of the World with the '7 Golden Rules of Zen Wisdom' with tools and techniques to help students in transforming them to leaders with social responsibilities.

"Ladies and Gentlemen, Put your hands together for Mr. Martin, a true gentleman."

"Mr. Martin walks up to the stage to accept the award with flashing lights, photographers and press reporters applauding his tremendous feat!"

With the flashing cameras, Martin's thoughts were back to a few decades earlier, reminiscent in his memories of Dr. Richard.

●●

Potraying The 7 Golden Rules of Zen Wisdom:

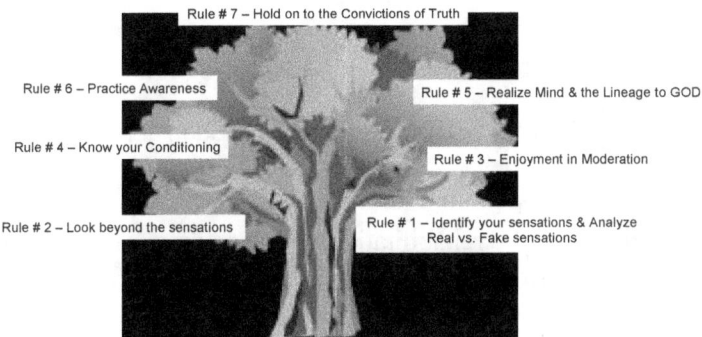

Rule # 7 – Hold on to the Convictions of Truth

Rule # 6 – Practice Awareness

Rule # 5 – Realize Mind & the Lineage to GOD

Rule # 4 – Know your Conditioning

Rule # 3 – Enjoyment in Moderation

Rule # 2 – Look beyond the sensations

Rule # 1 – Identify your sensations & Analyze Real vs. Fake sensations

The above WISDOM tree portrays the '7 Golden rules of Zen Wisdom'. As you progress in each of these steps, you'll be able to achieve the desired results and success in every endeavour you make. You'll need to practice it diligently.

'The 7 Golden Rules of Zen Wisdom' is an invitation to the contemporary men and women, who are brave enough to venture into the inner frontiers of Mind. It is an approach to reach the abyss of your mind by realizing the values of life. You have been procrastinating it for centuries and for lives together. The soul is hankering for the eternal '**TRUTH**', whilst the outer bodily/physical form is asking for more sensory pleasures.

You have the opportunity right now in transforming addictions to the audictions of truth, to grow spiritually by analyzing the '7 Golden Rules of Zen Wisdom'.

1

Dealing with Emotions

Mr. Martin was trembling – a sudden nervous breakdown gripped him, he was unconscious. The ambulance carried him to the rehabilitation centre to diagnose his condition. He was in a critical state with a dropping pulse rate.

The next morning he woke up in Dr. Richard's Rehabilitation centre with the doctor examining his condition.

"You'll be fine. Just get some rest," said the Dr. flashing his report.

Mr. Martin works as a Store Manager in a large retail store in Miami.

A few months later Martin relocates to South Carolina, and he visits Dr. Richard's rehabilitation centre in the downtown, South Carolina.

"Good Morning Madam!"

"Good Morning! responsed Dr.'s assistant, Becky."

"I would like to meet Dr. Richard."

"Welcome Mr. Martin! I hope you have an appointment?" asked Becky."

"Of course, I do. I called you last week from Miami! Thank you!"

Dr. Richard interrupts....

"Is that you? Martin from Miami!"

'Yes Dr., I am Martin from Miami. You had treated me in the Miami Medical Centre.'

"Oh boy!!! I remember. Miami. It's a beautiful place. I visit the Miami Medical Centre every month. You were very critical!"

"Well. How can I help you?"

Wearing a nice blazer and watching with blue sparkling eyes through his spectacle, Dr. Richard in his fifties started the discussions in his professional style.

"You can hang the coat there," he pointed to the hook.

He kept talking while walking towards the French window, to switch the lights for his patient.

Dr. Richard is a lovely gentleman, and a psychiatrist who has a record of treating his patients with extreme care and responsibility. He was raised in Milwaukee and settled in South Carolina. He conducts frequent workshops for his clients, all over the World.

"Can I get some coffee for you, Martin?"

"Yes Please," Martin says with a smile.

Dr. Richard asked his attendant to make two cups of nicely brewed Java café.

"How have you been since the last round of discussions my dear friend?"

Martin likes this discussion, seeking advice from Richard's generosity, and he started opening up a bit more than usual, after the first couple of meetings.

"Did I embarrass you?" asked Martin.

"I heard one of your councelling sessions, broadcasted last Friday in the CNN."

15

"Oh, you're talking about the '7 Golden Rules of Zen Wisdom'. Isn't it?"

"Yes Dr."

"Yup. That was grand success in the CNN. It was broadcasted on over fifty countries in the World. I've been getting calls from different regions to conduct workshops frequently. Unfortunately, I have less bandwidth and team to support a large Global programme."

"Well. That's exactly why I am here Dr."

"I'll need your help!!!!"

"Sure, I can help you. You'll need to go through the fourteen sessions as part of the workshops."

Martin agreed, with his greying hair reminding of his ageing. Martin in his early forties with strands of stress taking a toll in his forehead, and his neatly gelled hairstyle reminding of the 'James Bond-007', with the puzzled look on his face raising his eyebrow often as he speaks!

"Dr. Listen. Off late, I am not going through the trauma as often as I did!"

"Well. That's a fantastic progress." Dr. acknowledged.

"Perhaps, not with the same frequency. I do go through it occasionally."

"I would like the basic tests and details of your addictions prior to the workshops."

"Sure Dr."

"Please meet me with the ECG report and the case history details of your condition next week for the workshops."

"I suggest you continue with the medications until the workshops. Will discuss further by next week."

The following week:

"Well. Mr. Martin, that is certainly a progress."

With the documents, evidence of Martin's ECG analysis and brain scan test results. Now, it is late in the evening. Doctor was ready to leave the office carrying all his patient's profile to home.

"Bye." Martin started whispering with a sigh of relief.

Dr. Richard was surveying his patient's profile to find the recent historical records; he flipped through individual records and he stumbled on this one for Mr. Martin's case study in specific:

At times I feel hankering for sex, my brain gets heated up with my heart beating faster. Off late, I have started taking self-medication to reduce the body temperature.

I cannot sleep well during this excited state of my condition. I keep hankering for it. I try to focus on my work, but nothing would stop me until the point my animal instincts subside. Once I accept this, the next day my consciousness is guilt ridden. I go to the church pleading guilty, intensively to regain the lost energy, and praise the lord and surrender. This condition prevails for years now, perhaps for a decade, and I need medical assistance!!!

I am from a much respected family and have been following virtues as a practicing Christian, never had any particular instance ever in my life of any misdemeanor. I need help!!! Is there any medication available, or do I need to be admitted in a hospital for some time for psychiatric treatment? Am I addicted?

Only during these days my mind seems to be going haywire? I have a split personality as I guess. I am unable to live peacefully as my split mind is causing pain and guilt, and at times I want to commit suicide. When I regain confidence, the thought will disappear!

"What is my true situation Dr.? Did I repress my emotions? Am I addicted? Why is it happening to me alone? Can I get over such a condition and become a leader? I am successful in my job as a Store Manager. I am afraid of this negative behaviour with its consequences; I am well over thirty years of age, and need help as I lead a decent social life; It takes almost a week to get rid of the conditioning; I realize this is a particular conditioning."

Dr. Richard realized the conditioning was an "**Addiction**" as highlighted in the journal of psychiatry. Perhaps it was not properly diagnosed by the medical community he thought to himself, reading through the rest of the patient's case study.

Dr. Richard thought; without a doubt, this conditioning is an addiction. The impulsive behaviour is a specific situation as he formulated therapy techniques to help him out of addiction. Dr. Richard is not just a clinician, but also a practitioner of Zen meditation techniques with extensive knowledge in the Eastern Philosophy.

Often you go through the emotions of the mind in a state of excitement, anger or a sexual passion. Perhaps you'd dislike it in a guilt ridden consciousness then. How often has it happened to you? Perhaps right now you are going through some of these emotions, without resolving the conflict.

Dr. continues…

"Martin, your condition is not critical, however you'll need to go through the therapy sessions planned. In fact, I'd call it as techniques and tools to help you succeed in life."

"It sounds like a martial art". He looks around pictures of the Zen art everywhere in the centre.

"Yes. It does. But, the techniques that I am going to teach you is not physical, it is mental. It will help you change your perceptions and alter your priorities to succeed."

'Thanks Dr.!' Martin responded like a kid back to school to learn the techniques.

Let's start with the basic analysis:

"Do you manage your senses?"

"Managing what?" I didn't get that!

"Do you observe how the senses play the spoil sport?"

"Uh ….I haven't thought about that."

"Ok. Let me tell you something…"

Look at this formula:

Happiness Quotient (HQ) = KYS+LBS+EM ………….(1)

     Identify Your Sensations (IYS)

     Look Beyond the Sensations (LBS) and

     Enjoyment in Moderation (EM)

Realization Quotient (RQ) = KYC+RMLE+PA+HCT …(2)

     Know Your Conditioning (KYC)

     Realize Mind and Lineage to Eternity (RMLE)

     Practice Awareness (PA) and

     Hold on to the Convictions of Truth (HCT)

These are simple acronyms to memorize. It will help you succeed as you progress in the workshops.

'Ok. In first three topics, you'll be analyzing your senses, and I'll teach you how to manage your senses to get over your addictions, which is the formula for the Happiness Quotient (HQ).'

"Great. Thanks Dr!"

"In the last four topics, you'll know the roots of conditioning in mind and its lineage to eternity, which is the formula for the Realization Quotient (RQ).'"

"Interesting."

"Fasten your seat belts onto learn something very exciting, which will change your life forever, Martin."

19

Martin, you will need to practice these exercises discussed post the session, and contemplate deeply to understand the profound techniques. I've conducted these sessions all over the World to benefit over millions of students, entrepreneur to transform to great leaders.

You'll be transformed to a great leader by the end of the 14th Session. There is Q & A planned at the end of every session to answer all queries that you may have.

"Thanks Dr.!" Martin is prepared to learn once again, back to school. The real school of Altruism!!!

Day 1 - Session # 1:
Identify Your Sensations (IYS)

Write down ten emotional state of your mind. Analyze, when and where you are going through these situations. If you're feeling happy, feel thankful for the moment and just watch out. If you feel sad, and depressed, just observe. These emotions can inflict pain as they result in a negative mood such as depression; just be aware. It results in a deep state of negativity imported to your Mind, which will close the pores of the heart.

My perception is that your emotions are drained by the deep conditioning in the subconscious. You feel disturbed, when each of these emotions surfaces to the consciousness. The idea has been deeply rooted somewhere, eventually resulting in the emotions, behaviour and a repetitive pattern. This would result in an impulsive disorder or addictions. You must realize emotions closely, and its negative consequences in order to balance and restore the emotional well-being.

When you say that you are in an emotional state of mind, it can be beneficial or awful. This state of positive or negative emotions will require analysis. For instance: anger may be impulsive. It will subsidize over a period of time based on the analysis. You will be surprised to find each of these emotions is created by you, as it is all emerging deep from the subconscious mind.

As Sigmund Freud says every trauma at childhood, causing an impact at an adult age is a known fact. Your childhood fears of demons, ghosts can possibly subject you to fear even now as an adult or phobia of darkness is a result of the conditioning in the childhood. It is there as a conditioning deep down in the unconscious mind. When the situations reveal, you would project these imprints in mind. These are also known as karmic influences in the Eastern philosophy.

You will need to be aware of each of these emotions, analyze if it is causing pain or pleasure. How would you do it if you are in the emotional state of mind? Well, it is imperative to understand the excited state of mind. Mind is Nature's manifestation, and a gift to the human consciousness to realize the self and blossom to the fullest.

The purpose of life as stated in the Eastern philosophy is to recognize the underlying consciousness. It is the source of Mind, and reaching its core of consciousness by transcending the emotional state of Mind. '**The other end of Mind is GOD**'. The expanded state of Mind is GOD. It is all true, unless you learnways to transcend these emotions. These emotions will teach you if you get closer in research, instead of shying away and fearing them.

Each of you has quanta of all six temperamental moods inherited from the Genetics. It is an instinctive animal behaviour, in the evolutionary process. Now, God has endowed you with mind. It can be turned-in, and realize each of these emotions through a state of awareness to transcend, and realize the uninterrupted bliss. God has endowed you with the mirror called "Mind" to realize, and transcend negativity.

The emotions, sensations are all trading through the Mind. The Mind is in a constant traffic, isn't it? Often we ask others:

'How are you feeling today, Martin?'

"I am fine Dr., Thanks!"

'Perhaps, you have not asked the same question to yourself, to understand the underlying feelings. I believe you are aware of the Emotional Intelligence. This is the way you perceive and react forms your own behavioural pattern. The moods are subjective to changes based on the situation. What is the way out? Let us trace the emotions, feelings and the neurons that carry a certain impact in you. The root causes of negative emotions, and the penultimate responsibility to change the way you have been thinking, and feeling about yourself.'

Dr. Richard shows a Golden plate with a Rule embossed on it, here you go:

Rule # 1 – Identify Your Sensations (IYS)

'How do you deal with these emotions?' Wouldn't it be really nice, if an angel can elevate you with the sorcerer stone? It is none other than "YOU", who can transcend as the messiahs can only give you the roadmap. You will need to take the trail to succeed. Indeed, it is possible. You should have the desire to transform the mundane pleasures into eternal bliss. And extraordinary instances of pain, to circumstances of psychological growth. Let us explore these possibilities.

The below wheel of emotions as described by Robert Plutchik. You feel happy, excited at times, feel tender, scared, angry and sad many times. Each of these states eflects the fluctuations in your mind; or rather determine the 'moods', resulting in feelings of sadness or pleasure.

How do you conserve energy to succeed in life? Unless you get over your addictions, which are draining the energy. This is your integral part of being.

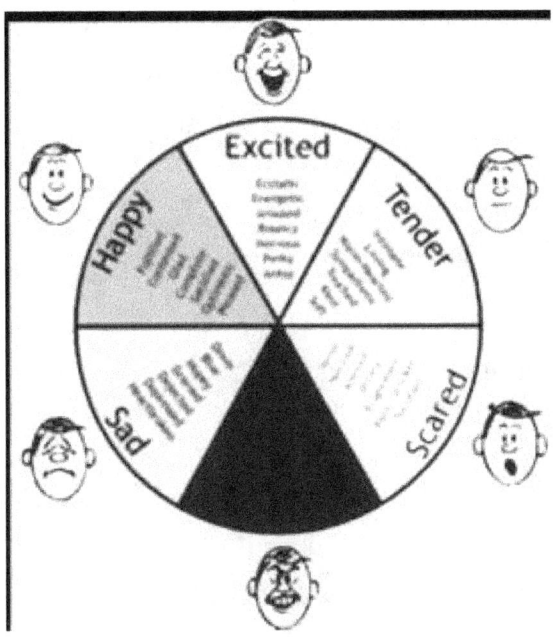

Dr. Richard had a plan to use profound therapy techniques to help him in the predicament.

"Ok. Martin, you will need to be here every weekend for the therapy sessions. I've planned for fourteen sessions."

"Ok. Dr." Martin responded.

They both walked into the therapy hall which was designed for talking to the soul as it looked with the soft white light and the couch that was made for comfortable relaxation.

"Here you go, Martin. Please lay down comfortably on the couch," he pointed out.

Dr. showed him a cyclic pattern to focus for a while and then instructed him to…

"Close your eyes," he indicated him to follow the instructions…

"Ok. Dr." Martin responded in a mild voice.

"I am gonna count from Ten to One, and follow me!"

"Take five deep breaths. In and out slowly and deeply."

"Now, Focus your attention between the eye-bro's and follow the sensations."

Then, he began counting TEN, NINE, EIGHT…relax, relax your body, mind and soul. And he continued to indicate SEVEN, SIX, FIVE..relax your organs…

FOUR, THREE, TWO and ONE…now you are deeply relaxed and the subconscious mind is awake. He brought his subconscious mind to the state of alertness using a soothing music.

"Now you tell me, how do you feel today?"

"I feel good today," he responded.

Ok. Good. What are these sensations?

"I feel sensations of happiness."

He asked questions in the flow of his hypnotic therapy. Then both were in sync, Q & A's started flowing in seamlessly well.

Now, You're back to the early stages of struggle. And pay attention, a little closer to the sensations.

"Of course Dr.," he was liaising with the depressed state of mind.

"Remember. You are just observing."

"Ah..Ok, Ok..Dr."

He then started crying as he started talking in a feeble voice, a little shaken.

"My relationships, breakups, addictions etc."

"Of course, it is painful," he concurred.

"Now pat you Martin. You've come out very well."

He was consoled. And it continued for almost couple of hours in going through the varying sensations of pain and pleasure.

"Well. Martin, we are towards the end now."

"Didn't you see the point of sensations?"

"What?"

These sensations of pain or pleasure are fluctuating. Didn't you realize these sensations?

"Absolutely Dr. I am able to identify these sensations."

"Very good! Catch them all," he expressed lovingly and passionately to his client.

End of Session # 1

Day 1 – Session # 2:
Analyze Your Sensations (AYS)

Let's get a little more closer analysis of your sensations. Have you pondered if all these sensations are real?

Ok. Let's have some chinese food before we discuss in detail.

"Ok. Dr."

"It's a nice cuisine, isn't it Martin?"

"Yes Dr."

"May I take the order sir?"

"Chinese Chicken Fried Rice! Dr. is busy in messaging to one of his clients."

"After a pause, Mr. Martin is ordering for a Chicken Soup!"

"I just had my lunch Dr. I am fine!"

"Good Job!" Dr. exclaims!!!

Dr. Richard was thinking about Martin's response as a good start as Martin is not just excited about food. Instead, his sensation was real!!! However, Dr. decides to testify him in another instance in the evening post the first session.

25

Did you understand it now? You are a writer, writing a script and a director of a movie called your '**LIFE**'. And everything manifests based on your **KARMAS** from the childhood till date. Everything that you have realized is all your emotions stored within as strands of the DNA. May be you have attracted it, and the spouse is the nearest reflection of the self! And your children are the closest reality.

The Divine Nature conspires through people around you. Therefore, "**YOURSELF**" should be the first level of analysis. Perhaps there is no need to criticize anyone else. Infact, you should be grateful to people around you, who have revealed the weakness, by helping you realize the conditioning in you. These neighbors, friends are the ones whom you have attracted by the karmic-debts, and they are postmasters of the Divine Nature.

The Divine Nature conspires everything through the fellow human beings. You have to learn from every incident in the life. It has an immense value if you understand and grow from the fact of life. For an example. If your spouse provokes anger, you should be grateful to her for helping you find emotions of 'anger', hidden in the abyss of the subconscious mind.

GOD has manifested as mind-wave. You will be able to recognize the divine consciousness mind in a subtle state of mind. The first step is to be aware of the '**EMOTIONS**' and let the light heal you. When you start observing each of these emotions, it will subdue. And further self-inquiry will guide you towards the centre of the inner self, where the purest state of consciousness resides. You have to understand self first, as the Divine manifestation of Nature. And there is nowhere to go, and no one to ask.

As Christ said:

"Knock the doors; Thou will open it for you."

When you knock the layers of the mind, the heart opens which is nothing but a subtle state of Mind where consciousness will reveal. Unfortunately, the mind is spinning in the sensations; addicted through the senses in six temperamental moods. Hence, you lose awareness frequently. The whole life has been conditioned from schools to the Universities without learning ways to seek truth through the inner revelations of consciousness based on self-inquiry.

The science has taught you examining and investigating the hypothesis in research! However, there is no examination of the mind to find the real self and the core of the consciousness. The Western school of thought or the education system is analysis based which involves scientific experiments to prove the hypothesis; whereas the Eastern school of mystic is based on the revelations of truth.

The heart centre is the centre of sensations, where you feel a little closer to the inner self and connected. These emotions are causing sensations of pain or pleasure; they are not real in many occasions as you may exclaim! When you think about a particular event, you'll be able to feel the sensations as it was happening just right now in the moment. The emotions are circular in nature as it is a wave, it will eventually end in the consciousness, as an impression of sensations within the centre of the self. Now, you have the ability to play back the sensations without having to confront a real situation. For example, think about any situation of the past, it will play back in mind, causing a similar sensation.

Only human mind can go back in time to retrieve an event to play back as thoughts. It looks so real! Now, the point is past sensations are not true at all; it is an excited state of the mind dissipating the magnetic energy (bio-magnetic wave). If it is so, then **what is a real sensation?** A real sensation is like when you are hit by a stone, and you would feel painful. This is absolutely true; You would still perceive a similar pain which is unreal while thinking about the events of the past. Most of us are just holding on to the past feelings of these cumulative sensations as pain.

I offered you lunch in the afternoon, which you denied. Did you see the point? You weren't feeling the sensations of hunger. Perhaps you could have been deceived by the senses with false sensations of hunger. However, You didn't want to relent yourself by having food or drink for camaraderie, isn't it? It indicates you weren't subjected to the external influences.

Good. Let's continue in next sessions.

The following week after the wonderful sessions, Martin was back on-time like a kid on-time to learn from the master.

"Ok. Martin, well done! Now, I am going to teach you something more exciting. Did you practice the session last week?"

"Yes Dr." Martin responded with a sense of responsibility and success.

"Martin, Didn't I tell you to catch these sensations in the last sessions?"

"Yes Dr. I did it too."

"Ok. Now, Pick up one of these sensations."

"I do have one." What is it?

"Dr., it is the most disgusting one…my addictions."

"Don't worry. It's fine. I'll help you to figure that out!"

"Now see through to identify the roots." What do you find? It's my craving. Can you explain, Martin?

"It's a craving for sex, Dr."

"Relax, don't be too serious. The bodily urge is natural!"

"Tell me, is it bodily urge or a mind thing?"

"Perhaps it is just a mind thing!"

"Ok. Martin. Where is it coming from?"

28

"Thoughts in Mind."

"Didn't you find the factor causing it, Martin?"

"Perhaps. My habits of watching pornography."

"Well. That's the point." He walked away with the lights on. Ok. Didn't you understand the sensations aren't real as it is created by you? And something in the backdrop of mind, creating it.

"Wouldn't you claim it as a false sensation?"

"Yes Dr. I would."

"I realize it now."

Dr. indicated, the purpose is to look beyond the sensations at the roots of it.

Rule # 1 – Identify Your Sensations and Analyze Your Real Vs. False Sensations (IYS and AYS)

The Real Vs. False Sensations

Once you gain experience of democrating between the Real Vs. False sensations, the False sensations will just fade away. I believe half of the problems will be resolved right now if you can distinguish between the Real Vs. False sensations.

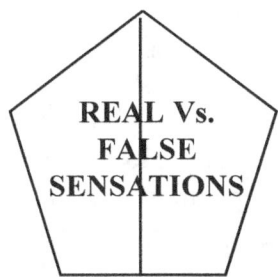

Now, Let us examine the imotions emerging from the subconscious mind.

The Emotional Bubble Burst

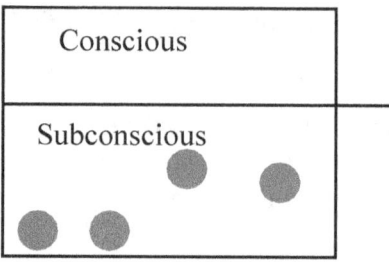

All of the emotions in the subconscious mind will emerge to the conscious mind. I intentionally drew the split with more space in the subconscious half, as more stuff is there without your knowledge.

You need to visualize the effects of an emotion. How painful it was? Or may be how much you've assumed it as happiness ending up in a disappointment. You need to contemplate to counsel and agree within yourself.

The self-experimentation will help you relieve from the painful sensations. You'll need to be alert the next day when the same situation occurs in seducing through the senses. It's like counselling a person "X" about harmful effects of smoking, which can result in diseases such as cancer. You will understand the importance of stopping unhealthy habits or addictions. You are empowering yourself through intellectual reasoning by exploring pro's and con's of an action. You aren't enforcing anything; instead you are revealing the facts in discreet terms by means of "**Monologue**" instead of a "**Dialogue**" within your subconscious mind by remaining as a witness.

The mind will be responsive enough to understand the consequences of negative karmic influences. You will be aware of it along with the consequences, which is useful. The above realization should extend to every action to recognize conflicting conditioning in Mind. You'll be able to comprehend the facts of consequences, every time the negative conditioning surfaces.

A simple analogy will help you understand. If you are smoking, the lungs are spoiled, and the doctor has advised about the harmful effect. You will remember the Doctor's advice, and the harmful behaviour with its consequences, everytime the urge starts. This is due to the fact that you remain a witness through practice. You have to draw a line between them and empower the positive thought to triumph over addictions.

Do you see my point; Mind will log in precision; hence, I'd like to call it as a tool, which will "**RECORD**" and "**REPLAY**" in precision. You have inflicted pain by imposing a negative condition; now, you have counseled yourself, narrating the harmful results of the behaviour such as "smoking". You will never be subjected to the negative condition as the positive condition will prevail along with it.

Remember, any act, thought in sync with Nature will have its lineage to the super consciousness Mind, and the opposite is true. This is the way to get rid of each of the conditioning; this exercise will increase the energy levels in meditation; The mind power should be used to examine the origin of mind, karmic-debts and progress in the journey of consciousness.

I have heard:

A Sadhu practices intense meditation in Himalayas.

God appears in front looking at his conviction.

"What do you want my son? You continue like a pauper by keep asking GOD."

"I want immense powers," he replied.

"Ok. So be it. You would gain powers as you wish to control the universe." As God granted powers to him. The demon goes on ransacking the towns, disturbing poor villagers, and angels!

Now, all angels pleaded to God to kill the demon; as God asked: "What is the matter?"

"My father, we are all being tortured," all other saints and angels pleaded to GOD.

GOD asks Chitra Gupta, "why is it so?" You are so humble at times of distress and if everything goes well, you seem to be have an inflated EGO subconscoiusness, that is not Natural.

The increasing money, fame, power and prestiege over will inflate the Ego, and it turns outwardly, indulging through the sensual pleasures. If you do not expand the mind, you will continuously hanker for one-hundred and one things! This is a Natural tendency. Your emotions have boundaries. It cannot transcend beyond the mundane pleasures. A new 'object' will give you pleasure for a couple of days, a new bike for hours, a new mobile phone for minutes until you find another one.

The above tendency of the mind has extended in the relationships too; as a beautiful date as-of last month, is no longer beautiful. The reason is that you cannot confine mind to the limits of boundaries, and you keep hankering for something more. No matter how much you enjoy through the sensual perceptions. Each of the senses has specific limits, and it cannot go beyond the limitations. On the contrary, your Mind has infinite potential, and it is a natural desire to reach its organic unity. It is like a river finding the Ocean!!! It's an orgasmic unity, and the mind is a microcosmic truth which would like to merge with the macrocosmic reality!

As a result, the inner mind wants more, and more and you can only feed its urge by merging with the infinite consciousness. If emotions are confined to the boundaries, you will keep circling like a tamed lion; going on in circles. The entire Universe is there for you to explore, from the mountains to the valleys. The beautiful rivers, and Oceans. You have to realize the wonders around you!!!

The ultimate urge is to unite with the eternal being itself, to feel the orgasmic unity in eternity. Your senses are bound by the limitations. You cannot drive a passenger car at thousand miles, whereas it is possible in an aircraft, and even more so in the rocket engines cranking at more than thousand miles/hr. Mind has infinite capacity, which cannot be confined to the sensual perceptions alone.

If you are attracted by the senses, constantly you will over indulge based on the natural urge, which becomes a habit eventually. The 'urge' was a need perception created by Nature for you to transcend, and progress towards the journey of consciousness into eternity. It is a minimal taste of the macrocosmic truth. In my view, each of it has a quality. In the beauty itself from the fragrance of flowers to the eyes of a woman!

This is a 'LEELA' or a vicious cycle in life. Perhaps a litmus test. If you do not climb, you will never grow spiritually. You should understand, and live life to the fullest and the transformation of mundane life into uninterrupted blissfulness, which is possible by transforming miseries in the happiness. There seems to be no rationale in anything you do. May be you seem to be truly humble in the beginning, until you succeed in the mundane World.

The "EGO" is an excited state of MIND. Perhaps it is a hallucination in mind as it does not exist; 'Mind is a WAVE'. And it is conditioned based on the baseline personality. May be you've observed examples of sixteen factors attribute to the baseline personality.

The mind has to turn inward by focusing on the source itself to realize its lineage to GOD. The source of mind is life-force, and the centre is consciousness, which is eternal. You'll be sooner or later bored by going through the sensory perceptions alone, forgetting the lineage to the eternity. This is the ultimate secret! God wants you to learn from the experiences, sensations and the enjoyment within limitations and transcend to the centre; by finding the core without any repressions.

You have to be sensitive to the feelings as discussed, there is a natural desire to sublimate. If you repress, you will become a pervert. The spiritual path of transcendence is to sublimate it by proper means by aligning yourself to the laws of Nature. The path of Yoga is the balancing act by using the senses with utter responsibility.

"Everything seems to be perfect

Except my conditioned Mind!"

When I opened up my heart by realizing the 'FALSE' sensations, I felt incessant flow of energy within myself; I would suggest dropping the False sensations right now as it is all illusionary. I am going to explain how '**Mind is an illusion**'. We'll go through the sensations first and understand emotions which are causing these sensations.

"Why are you feeling so depressed right now?"

I asked someone:

He said: "I did not get in to the college that I liked the most!" The same misery is drowning in someone as a lost love, or a lost car or may be a lost job! Whatever it is subject to degree of attachment to the object.

It is just a pattern. A real depression should be starvation as an exception; These are the real needs for survival. If you are not able to fulfil the needs, then there is a definite reason to feel depressed, which is a natural desire to sublimate basic instincts. I'd summarize in simple terms all righteousness is manifestations of the Divine Nature. You feel dissatisfied on particular events, ideas, circumstances based on the baseline conditioning. If it results as per your calculations, you are perfectly happy; any detour is creating anxiety in you. However, Nature has other plans. He is eternally merciful, in a way he is ruthlessly honest as he reveals it by means of "**CAUSE and EFFECT**" theory, which is reaping up the benefits of what you've sown. May be you have inherited the **KARMAS** as "**GENETICS**"

34

through the parents, and ancestors. I am not blaming you for all the negative emotions. May be encouraging you to look beyond a particular event or events or a set of people.

These are all the post-masters who are carrying the Divine FACET to you based on the past conditioning. Perhaps you will react by yelling at a pizza boy for delivering pizzas late. Often you haven't realized the background story of a Pizza boy, who tries hard to deliver, and he fails occasionally. You have to understand these emotions are the delivery mode of the past conditioning, resulting in sensations of pain or pleasure. You're bound to watching it helplessly.

The mind can cripple you, and rip your heart apart, based on the baseline analysis, which may be 'right' or 'wrong'. Perhaps your set of assumptions from the baseline analysis are invalid. You will need to change the assumptions to the "**Intellectual**" reasoning. You're wrong if these assumptions are from the conditioned mind. Therefore you miscalculate every single event, as a result, creating a major disaster; as each of these assumptions will turn sour over a period of time based on the actual results.

Well. Enough of beating around the bushes; what is the way out? When you have your own consciousness as the 'Boss', it will help you succeed in life. You have turn one hundred and eighty degrees, turning yourself to the centre of the consciousness.

'**What else do you want?**' If the emotions are in sync, with the sensations and thoughts etc. The mind will be in the ultimate state of blissfulness, and ecstasy enjoying the Divine Nature in the moment to moment awareness as portrayed in the Zen stories. Now, you are familiar with the art of segregating between your "Real" Vs. "False" Sensations, and practice it diligently.

"Well done!" Dr. congratulates Martin for learning the Rule # 1. You've mastered the first rule is simple, let's remember this:

Rule # 1- Identify Your Sensations and Analyze Your Real Vs. False Sensations (IYS and AYS)

Now, the second rule is to look beyond these sensations that are inflicting pain in you. He shows the Golden plate with the second rule embossed on it.

End of Session # 2

Day 2 – Session # 3:
Look Beyond Tthe Sensations (LBS)

After a couple of phenomenal sessions, Martin was even more enthusiastic to learn the art of transformation, and Dr. Richard glowing in his sparkling eyes with a glass of wine.

"Toast. My dear friend," he hugged Martin for the success session.

The mayor has invited me for a dinner! He wanted me to interview Mr. President. "That's a real good news, Martin said, tasting the Italian wine."

"You've passed the first two sessions, now the third one is very simple."

"What is it Dr.?"

Ok. You have picked the 'Sensations', and then analyzed "Real" Vs. "False" Sensations as you did in the first session. In the second session, you realized the cause of it!

Rule # 2 - Look Beyond the Sensations (LBS)

Did you realize some of these negative emotions are creating an impulsive behavioural pattern? You have become victims without knowing what to do! There is a temporary relief by taking some alcohol or perhaps medications to soothe your neurons. It numbs the perceptions temporarily!

36

Look at the mind circle below that depicts your fluctuating mind in varying sensations.

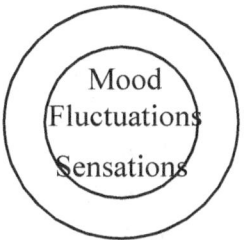

Let me ask you a question **"Did addictions have helped you solve anything?"** Obviously not. As I hear you all saying that unanimously! At least based on the artifacts, all inventions, discoveries have occurred in the subtle state of mind. You do not achieve anything in an aggravated state of mind. As a matter of fact, most crime happens by the seductive nature of mind. The mind-wave will replay imprints through the brain cells in neurons as perceptions with a chemical reaction. It is all well-coordinated through the autonomous nervous system.

There is no need to be antagonistic against anything...not even your negative or positive sensations. Perhaps these are sensations that are creating an awareness in you. To be deep rooted in you with the emphasis: "who the real "you" are!

You should look beyond the sensations in realizing the origin. Perhaps you might be in a depressed state of mind or an elevated state! Whatever the case, write it down and contemplate. The fluctuations in Mind are on the periphery whilst sensations are in the core of the being. Aren't you feeling the consequences from external circumstances? The outer affects the inner and vice versa.

These sensations are all a state of flux, retrieved from the subconscious mind, causing sensations. It is imprinted in each of you, and replayed back when you want to retrieve one by one when you remain silent. Hence, the chaos and chatter in Mind.

Did you realize, Nature has not created human consciousness overnight; it is an evolutionary process over millions of years of cumulative experiences that eventually develop the human consciousness. Just imagine the marvel of mind with the capacity to think, rationalize, memorize, and expand to the infinite. Is it not a wonder! What is the idea of the evolution of mind endowed with human consciousness? I strongly believe there is a purpose. Indeed Nature has created your mind to analyze. To help you understand the sensations – **Emotions – Feelings - Thoughts** and **Conditioning**. And finally realize the purest consciousness at the centre itself as its manifestations.

GOD wants you to realize, based on your own understanding, with the revealing events. He knocks the door in the morning sun shine. The chirping birds are singing everyday to wake you up. Here, it is a trick, **how do you realize mind as the manifestations of Nature?** The mother Nature has created everything in a state of subtle frequency. A specific attunement of the mind is required. This indicates the responsiveness to practice in order to realize the wonders of Nature. A simple analogy is like tuning an FM RADIO. Nature will reveal all secrets one-by-one in a subtle state of pure mind.

Do you realize the bottom of sensations? Who realizes the pain or pleasure? Each of these sensations will result in dissipating the energy through mind; These sensations are like waves in the Ocean. It represents a state of flux in the mind. It is like striking a chord of a guitar; perhaps if you strike it correctly it will create a rhythm called incredible music, else it will be chaotic, isn't it?

The experiences are imprinted as sensory perceptions, which is repetitive and you play it back wrongly. You would find achorus going haywire, isn't it? The same is true; if you use your mind incorrectly, you are stuck to it forever and the cycle continues. God never wants you to go on in circles; perhaps he wants you to enjoy through the senses in sensory perceptions that are the reason why you have five senses and the sixth sense: Finally the ultimate "**MIND**" has evolved in the human beings, to perceive its own potential, and its lineage to the Nature.

There is nothing wrong in the enjoyment as that is the objective of God, providing you the senses. Only you're thinking of overdoing it in an indulgence is the cause of all problems in life. It is due to either innocence or ignorance. I believe '**Ignorance is bliss**' is true in children; however, it cannot be justified in adults. If a cop pulls you over for reckless driving, would you argue that you were not aware of the driving rules? You cannot have an excuse for not learning! It is your responsibility to learn the skills to drive it with safety.

Alright. Over consumption of alcohol is giving you a sensation of "pleasure". All I am saying is that, you should look beyond the pleasure into the facets of sensations that are causing it. You'll find these false sensations are caused by numbing the neurons. It blocks the nerve centre Vs. organ coordination and impairs the ability to think. If you watch closely, the consumption of alcohol enters into the blood stream, and slows down the process of thinking by numbing the capacity to respond to the environment. Hence, you start projecting, and it looks so real! You fantasize and the reality seems too far away from the heart! In the next morning, you'll have to face the real life situations, which becomes a bigger challenge! You didn't get any closer to solving your problems.

A simple analysis as above has yielded you to think beyond the sensations. You should try to analyze these sensations to identify the roots. Once you capture the roots of it, it will be easy to change the core perceptions. None can deny the responsibilities that each one of you carry! You often forget the theory of Cause and Effect, and then repent after an action yielding negative impact. Indeed mind should govern these senses to evolve through consciously. There is no need to forsake anything in the name of spirituality.The third session had started. A little intense, and starting to the point."

"Martin, didn't you realize the sensations of pain?"

"Yes Dr. I looked beyond the sensations of pain, these are created when I go over the board."

"Like what, Martin. Please explain."

"Dr. When I drink little, It is more relaxing. When I exceed a certain limit, I create all problems, as I start projecting my desires."

"True. I've heard from the bartenders while investigating your drunken behaviour," Dr. chuckles.

"Alright. How do you realize, when you exceed the limits and who states it to you?"

Perhaps you should realize it, Dr. continued talking about the enjoyment in moderation. The sensation of happiness turns sour, when you exceed the limits. Let me ask you something...

"Here is the Italian spaghetti and sausage with wine served right now."

"Ooohh..that's my favourite food. I am very pleased Dr. Richard."

"Wait a minute." Eat it slowly. Let's start.

As Dr. kept talking intentionally, analyzing his behaviour. Martin has crossed the limits and he started feeling a little uncomfortable sensations. Another serving, another drink, please.

"Ok. Sure" Martin continued...

And finally, he couldn't take it anymore. He puked.

"Oooops. I am sorry!"

"That's ok. Now, relax for a while. I would like to emphasize on enjoyment in moderation. Didn't you realize?"

"Yes, I do, Dr." Martin acknowledged his behaviour.

"Let's talk about the 'Enjoyment in Moderation'."

End of Session # 3

Day 3 – Session # 4:
Enjoyment in Moderation (EM)

Have you observed all these sensations are limited to boundaries? These senses have boundaries as you cannot go beyond a certain level of entertainment; For example, Would you be able to listen to the favourite music for hours? You will get tired after a while; It is due to dissipating your own energy as a conversion through the senses. The net loss of energy will be compensated in sleep as per Nature's plan. These sensations are quanta of bio-magnetic energy converted; when it exceeds a specific limit, that is where all problems starts, and you get addicted to the senses!

Perhaps you would like to have a sumptuous Italian dinner with little Italian wine. This is absolutely rejuvenating as you recall, and you started enjoying food to the core. After another serving of chicken sausage with parmesan cheese, may be you feel a little more filled. And one more serving! A few moments ago, the sumptuous, mouth-watering food served was delightful to the senses. This sensation has turned upside down and now you feel like jumping out of the restaurant, isn't it?

"What happened to you Martin?" asked Richard.

"I felt heavy and uncomfortable sensations in my stomach!"

"Weren't you enjoyed the same food and wine served a little while ago?"

"Of course, I did!"

A simple logic..If one serving is rejuvenating to your senses, perhaps two servings should multiply your sensations of happiness, isn't it?

Martin agreed to Dr. Richard's point of view. They both were listening to a music.

Beck is Dr.'s assistant. "Becky, could you increase the volume, please." She responded quickly, and threw the remote control to Dr. "Here, you go!"

"Thanks Becky!" Dr. caught the remote. He then continued to increase the volume to a loud music. Almost the entire floor was resounding like a dance floor.

"Shake it, shake it, move it, move it."

"How do you feel, Mr. Martin?"

"Perhaps, I feel like dancing."

"Then, go-ahead." Dr. pointed out to the mini-dance lounge where Beck was listening.

"Becky, would you like to take the floor by storm?"

"Yes," she responded. They both danced for a while.

After an hour, Dr. interrupted. Let's continue!!! He started increasing the volume to the maximum possible.

Martin interrupted. "Excuse me, Dr. Richard. It's too loud, would you please stop it?"

"Why don't you dance? It's exciting." Dr. tried to explain.

"No, sorry. I cannot do it anymore." Martin replied.

"Well. Well. This is the point of elasticity. Dr. explained the graph indicating how the pleasure, turning into pain. You should know it even before it happens. You gotta be smart my dear friend."

Becky acknowledged him with a smile, having seen Dr. Richard's intelligence for almost a decade now.

"Yes Dr. I hear that." Martin responded.

So the purpose is to "Enjoy in Moderation." You were enjoying it till the point of elasticity. Beyond that, it turns sourly. Now, you'll need to analyze in moods of food, rest, work, intercourse and thoughts to stay within limits. Each of it will deplete your mind-power if you exceed the limits.

"Ok. Dr., I'll practise it." Martin walks out of the tenth floor thinking about the session.

It is a simple logic if one serving could offer you 'x' amount of happiness, and logically two servings should perhaps give you 'x+1' happiness. Unfortunately, the 'Laws of Nature' is diametrically opposite. If you over do it, it becomes 'X-1'!!! Hence, you feel the reverse sensations of happiness, turning into a depression.

A real entertainment through the senses turns as a virtual pleasure as 'thoughts'. You'll be able to replay these sensations as it records precisely and replays it back like a CD player. These sensations are fictitious, rather than the actual sensations. You might have observed, the moment you think about the experiences, it comes with the sensations of pleasure, or pain as a memory. Perhaps you are addicted to the virtual sensations through the mental phenomena, rather than a real thing, in the process of thinking.

This will result in all sorts of mental disorders, eventually affecting the body. The sensory entertainment should be in moderation. If you exceed the limits, it becomes a pain as I had stated. It is not renouncing anything you have joyously accepted a bowl of soup, a cup of tea. It is essential, and the fundamental aspect to follow if you want to live a healthy and peaceful life.

Some people do learn from the mistakes; they recover quickly, and some repeat their mistakes till the end of life, those who are ignorant. It happens despite several warnings by Nature, as they cross the bridge under repair, to free fall into a pit. These are all cumulative experiences you should try and learn from the mistakes and the lessons learnt, there is no point in repeating it over and over again.

The sensory enjoyment cannot last beyond a certain boundary. For example, you perceive through the senses, through the vision or ears listening to music, which can give you a certain pleasure.

Rule # 3 Enjoyment in Moderation (EM)

Did you analyze the way you perceive pain or pleasure?
There is an energy (bio-magnetic) circuit in the physique. This is a simple analogy of electricity circuit and the conversion through senses is observed by mind as a 'pain or pleasure'. If the unit spent through the senses is within a permissible limit of conversion, the mind translates it as 'pleasure' through the brain cells. On the contrary if you exceed the limits by abusing the senses, then it will cause a pain due to the short circuit, which is an interrupted flow of biomagnetism.

A simple analogy is the electricity. What is electricity?

It is a flow of electrons, isn't it? What is a short-circuit? If you interrupt the flow of electrons (electricity), it is called a short-circuit! Perhaps I'd try to get back to the basics that we learnt in the highschool.

Well. The short-circuit is caused by an external interruption; obstructing the flow. The same is true in the physiology; there is a circuit of energy (bio-magnetic) formed within the body. If the circuit is disturbed, then you'd end up in a disturbance as sensations of pain. If it persists longer, it is known as a disease. There is no point in treating the diseases in isolation as you are organically connected between body, mind and soul. If the essential flow of energy is disturbed, it will affect the body first and then mind and soul. The circuit in your body is altered due to excessive behaviour with the excessive dissipation of the magnetic energy beyond the acceptable level of conversion.

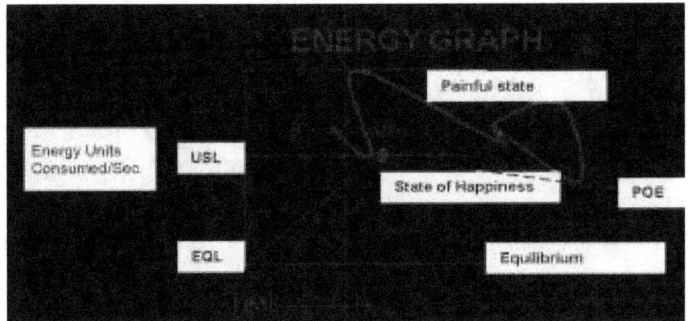

USL – Upper Specification Limit

EQL – State of Equilibrium

POE – Point of Elasticity

The above energy graph indicates the energy consumption/sec in the Y axis, and TIME in the X axis. As you continue to enjoy using senses, there is a USL – Upper Specification Limit that you'll need to adhere to maintain within limits. The section "A" is the area of happiness in mind. The section "B" is the area of painful state and EQL is the line of equilibrium state of mind.

If you exceed the limits of elasticity, as indicated above, the graph goes haywire in section B, which indiactes the painful state. The energy curve indicates the deviation from the Upper Specification Limit (USL), hence the consumption of energy units/sec is much higher than the equilibrium state. As a result, you'll deplete your conserved energy.

When you reach the point of elasticity, your senses MUST stop. If you exceed this limit, it becomes pain. The same sensations of happiness turns in to painful sensation. The Upper Specification Limit (USL) indicates the limits in moderation, if you exceed, it will turn painful. This logic applies to every sensual enjoyment.

Let's say in the above example. You were enjoying the food as you progressed; you overate causing nausea.

The sensations of pain or pleasure is all discharge of the energy circuit within your body. The energy circuit flows through the senses, here it is 'tongue', And it is transforming the energy into certain units of taste through the tongue. Three (3u) units of energy is the state of equilibrium in tounge, which is excited by an external stimuli-food to five (5u) units. The delta of two units is perceived by the mind as the sensation of pleasure. The tongue is capable of enjoying to the extent of about five (5u) units. Beyond a limit, it will alert the brain cells to stop behaving the way you are doing! Let us assume the state of elasticity limit is 10 units. If you exceed 10 units, the sensations of pleasure will turn to the sensations of pain.

God has endowed you with senses to enjoy by understanding its limits. It will message you, when you start exceeding. It is due to lack of awareness that you'll exceed. It becomes a habit. The graph will vary depending on the usage of your senses. The irony is that if you ignore the messages of the limitation of senses, it will lead to diseases. Each instance you exceed the limits, will have its consequences of altered cellular structure. Thus, it impacts your equilibrium state and discord in **BODY, MIND** and **SPIRIT**, resulting in long term diseases.

The above analogy will apply for all your sensory enjoyment such as food, rest, intercourse, work and thoughts. The above factors will need to be experienced in a state of awareness, to enjoy within limits, to maintain equilibrium. Hence, it is a social responsibility to analyze situations where you will exceed the limits. The subtle mind will try to convey it to the senses, due to the sensual pleasure when the limits are reached. Thereon, you have been forgetful without enjoying within limits...an excess would result in pain. Say in anything overeating causes diabetes at a later age, or perhaps extreme sexual addictions would result in diseases etc. This is an intrinsic plan of the Nature. Bhagvat Gita says 'Karma Yoga' and be totally aware of what you do. If you are aware, you'll not be subjected to the sensory peceptions alone. Your centre will indicate the point of elasticity in the sensory perceptions.

The authentic sensations like hunger, or sex is natural. It should not be repressed, and it is your responsibility to sublimate with proper means. These sensations are pleasant, but the way you choose to dissipate should be in liaison with the society and the laws of Nature, without causing any disharmony to the self or anyone.

The real virtue is the righteous means of dissipating real sensations without exceeding the limits. These laws are intrinsic, and the Universal Laws are governed by Nature. If you understand these fundamental laws of Nature and live in unison with it is a Divine act, and religious. There is no need to go to any temple, synagogue, or a church to understand this simple '**CAUSE and EFFECT**' theory. The real challenge is to understand it quickly at a young age, and synchronizing your activities with the laws of Nature.

Your inheritence is animal kingdom, and the basic instincts are Natural. The ultimate challenge is to realize the basic instincts and sublimate by striking a balance. The balancing act of body, mind and spirit is known as **Yoga**.

The compulsive behavioural pattern thus created in the Genetics will keep you entangled through the lifetime repercussions till the end with no benefit. Instead, if you socialize with these sensations through the way of meditation, and introspective analysis will transcend you to the next level of consciousness from the 'unconscious'reaction to the 'conscious' action. In fact animals are reflexive by Nature, you will be acting like an animal without being able to change the reflexive behaviour.

We have discussed the emotions, sensations and the roots of it; which is creating the sensations of 'good' or 'awful'. Also, we had enough discussions on the conditioning and addictions. I would like to discuss it in separate chapters on conditioning and social addictions, and the 'media' which has created the milieu in you. The moment someone pulls the strings of emotions, you would go bang all out till the end, venting it out! You are just awaiting a reason to vent out like a volcano steaming in and fuming in, when time comes you burst out, which is due to the conditioning. The strings of emotions have to be streamlined as you have analyzed the Actual Vs. Virtual. Now you know which ones to get rid of, and the ones which are authentic.

You can sublimate it by constant self-counseling, and deep realization as soon as you become aware of these emotions. If you are reactive to the circumstances, as often you'll find yourself in a state of the quagmire, without realizing unfolding events. You will just responding to the stimuli, with no control over life.

Hence, I request you to do things in totality; by consciously drinking tea, eating food or fetching water leaving no trace of mind. I realize that each of the conditioning is due to the lack of totality or a two dimensional view of events. When the event unfolds, and you regret about the past events, and you long for it once again, if it is good and detest for the negative emotions. Essentially the differences lay in the perceptions, and the way you respond to stimuli.

You've mastered the first three rules of The 7 Golden Rules of Zen Wisdom:

Identify Your 'SENSATIONS' (IYS);

Look 'BEYOND' the sensations (LBS);

Enjoyment in 'MODERATION' (EM).

End of Session # 4

2
Development Psychology

Day 4 – Session # 5:
Know Your Conditioning (KYC)

The fifth session was ecstatic as Martin started enjoying every moment.

"Martin, We will discuss the various facets of conditioning a little more deeply, and the behavioural pattern. You have realized the essence of "**SENSATIONS**" and the unfolding "**EMOTIONS**"."

You've realized the sensations, roots of it by looking beyond it, and enjoyment in moderation. Now, the fourth important point is to teach you **identifying** the conditioning in mind.

"What is a conditioning, Dr.?"

"Listen carefully. As you go through the workshop today, you'll get it."

"Ok. Dr." Martin responding with a sense of triumph.

"Didn't you find sensations of pain, pleasure are a kind of repetitive?"

Dr. continued talking, you have learnt the lessons of Sensations, Looking Beyond the Sensations and Enjoyment in Moderation. Now, its time to Identify the Conditioning. The most important session that I would like to teach you today!

"Ok. Dr." Martin responded like a student hungry for knowledge.

"Martin, let me ask you this."

"What is conditioning?"

"Dr. to be honest, I don't know."

"That's alright." I'll describe.

 "Do you believe in Christ?"

"Of course. I do."

"Can you explain?" Dr. asked.

"I was taught from my childhood to practice Christianity. It helps."

"Perhaps, you were taught in childhood."

"Yes."

"You were told that Heaven and Hell exist and if you follow Christ you would go to Heaven!"

"Yes."

"How do you prove this hypothesis?"

"Well. I just believe it."

"Ok." Did you believe it without realization out of the heart?

"Yes."

"This is one of the social conditioning."

"You saw everyone around you and influenced by their behaviour."

This is the first condition in mind as "Virtue" Vs. "Sin". The conditioning by the religion. I would call "The social conditioning" based on the blind faith. Every Religion has created a set of blind faith in the respective individuals as 'Virtues'.

Look at this… Dr. points out to the presentation:

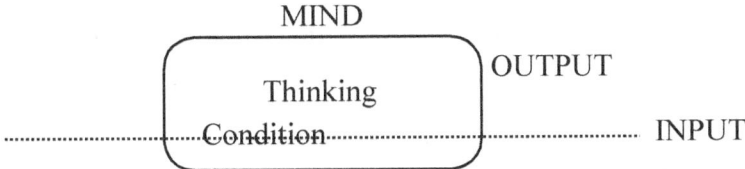

This is a conditioning. Your MIND in the centre responding to the INPUT in order to respond as an OUTPUT in the process of Thinking. For example,

"Why do you think Christianity or Hinduism or Islam is good?"

"Well. I was told Christ is the only 'Son of God.'"

"Perhaps, you were conditioned."

"Everytime you think about Christ, the output of your mind makes a statement: 'Christ is the only son of GOD' as you were conditioned in the subconscious mind. Did you get my point? It's not your revelations. It is your belief!

"Yes Dr." Martin responded.

You were reactive!

This is your point of view about Christ.

Hang in there. Let me call someone.

Krish walks into his office. "Welcome Krish!" Dr. Richard hugs him. Krish is a practicing Psychiatrist. He is brilliant.

Krish, can you walk through the facts of conditioning?

"Yes Dr." Krish started explaining…

You'll need to analyze the process of thinking with the conditioning in the backdrop. Perhaps you'll need to question each of the Conditioning in mind.

Rule # 4 Know Your Conditioning (KYC)

"Martin, could you write about emotions on the board please?"

"Sure," he walks to the board to write:

Pain	**Happiness**
Pleasure	**Bliss**
Truth	**Resentment**
Guilt	**Embarrassment**

These are all EMOTIONS in the mind.

GOOD JOB!!!

"Mr. Martin, as you ponder in each of these emotions, which reflect the state of being, isn't it?"

"Aren't you influenced by Christ?"

"Yes, I am."

One of the social conditioning influencing your ability to think. Well. "What is MIND?"

"Perhaps MIND is thinking!"

That's your view. You were influenced by the science classroom sessions.

"My view is different as a Psychiatrist."

"Ok. What about a simple math:

$(a+b)2 = a2+b2+2ab$....(1)

"Good Job! You still remember maths very well!!!!"

"True. I am a class topper in the highschool."

"Good. Can anyone deny the formula he just wrote on the board as incorrect?"

"It is a scientific derivation, and none can deny it."

"True. Another one $E=MC^2$". Can you challenge this one.. Einstein's theory of relativity?

It's scientifically proven too, why would anyone deny a formula.

"That's exactly correct, Mr. Martin."

"Your conditioning is all assumptions imposed on you by the society or family in the name of aset of conduct with limited reasoning."

"You are already setup for a failure by this conditioning in mind, unless you replace the condition with a formula, which is your own revelations."

"Dr. Please explain."

Krish continued . . .

"Ok. The society, media, internet and politics all explore sex as the fantasy. Did you examine the basics and roots of it?"

"Well. I didn't do till now."

"You get excited about everything, being reactive."

"True."

"You were conditioned" and influenced in everything you do from morning to evening.

Like a shaving gel that you're using is influenced by the famous actors in an advertisement. It was not your conscious choice to pick up the gel that you liked. You are not on your own. Just branded by these brands from Jean to the shoes that you were using is all conditioning. You're living like a brand ambassadors for someone! Didn't it make you feel better or betrayed by the social conditioning? You've completely lost your own identity as a result, as you're behaving like a noblest and the best actor on the stage.

"True Dr. I understand that now."

This is a beginning of a radical change in thinking, where you reflect on each of these emotions. May be a little more psychoanalysis to understand the situations that are causing them. Let's take a deep dive into the emotions deep in the subconscious mind revealing the inner treasures of life.

"Do you evaluate it as right or wrong?" Your ability to transform a particular event through intellectual reasoning and self-inquiry; The process of thinking involves evaluating the input, based on the events, and circumstances recognize it as 'GOOD' or 'BAD' in order to react to the environment accordingly. Here is the point. The evaluation is subjective to your analysis. How would you know it is right, unless it is a revelation from your won consciousness? The so called 'beliefs' cannot go deeper into the conscious mind if it is a belief based system imposed on you. In this case, the subconscious mind will succeed. If you realize the harmful conditioning through intellectual reasoning and inner revelations, the conscious mind will succeed!!!

All Gurus can give you revelation of their own. It is your practice and revelations of the inner self that will help. The karmic debts will be cumulative, unless you recognize the truth residing within you, it will keep you entangled. May be you haven't uncovered it so far.

These karmic influences will surface from the unconscious mind to the conscious mind, while you are observing '**SILENCE**'. Perhaps you can try it for a day and gradually increase to help you uncover the truth. These Universities have failed to teach the basics of human physiology, reproductive organs, or behavioural science. The social study is not helping you understand the basics of sociology, meditation, yoga etc. It has succeeded in creating mindless robots, but failed miserably in creating humans, in helping them in the evolution of consciousness. More so, minds have become addicted to the senses. The addictions are increasing with several disorders of modern times.

Once you read through the healing techniques, may be you can practice it regularly at work at it takes 15-20 minutes to reflect, combined with exercises. I have observed people point out 'WORK' as an excuse, without realizing the importance of analyzing your mind and its conditioning.

Ask yourself, "**Do you work to live or live to work?**"

If you are firm in what you want to achieve, actions will result as manifestations of the thoughts. If you honestly call the Divine in love and surrender yourself, you will find ways to collaborate with the like-minded people. And finally the microcosmic mind will attract the like-minded super-consciousness Divine Nature itself. Think about whom you want to be from now, a mediocre life transformed to the life of blissfulness in six months from now.

The below graph indicates your spritual growth as your grow bilogically.

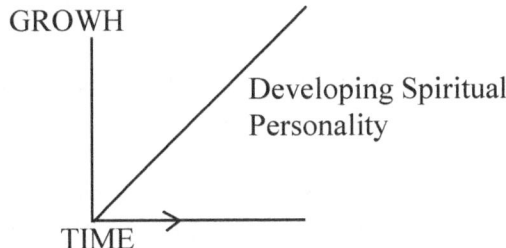

GROWH

Developing Spiritual Personality

TIME

"Mr. Martin, you've to prepare the schedule as typically we do before starting up a project plan on the board. Allow six months pass by as per the plan, evaluate the changes. Feel it and let the experience be the revelations of truth and feelings, emotions of pain, anguish and fear will melt away as you progress."

The inner consciousness will speak to you in absolute SILENCE, with your heart becoming lighter. There will be glimpses of bliss, which is your revelations of the heart. Your perspective will change, without hankering for anyone or any object, to be happy. The happiness will become your intrinsic quality with an uninterrupted bliss. You will be able to share the blissfulness with everyone by spreading the joy everywhere, in any confronting situation without being subjective to the emotional state of mind.

End of Session # 5

Day 5 – Session # 6:

Martin, don't you find the reason to identify your condition to succeed in all your endeavour? Let us analyze the basics of your conditioning as Zen portrays it as a prominent factor in the behavioural analysis.

Perhaps you should 'Stop being reactive'. Let's analyze anger as part of the analysis. Did you ever analyze the situations that are causing anger in you? Each of these emotions is not based on the circumstances. Do you think it is because of others or subjective to your inner self. As a matter of fact, your anger has always been there and it is not even provoked by the spouse, neighbors or even surroundings. Mostly, it is a condition in you which is causing all disaster. The point is "YOUR CONDITION" is responsible for all problems till now.

The split mind is a constant trouble; as the outer desires more, and the heart desires for eternal love. The facts are concealed by religion, and you are made a scapegoat by the religious leaders in the name of guilt ridden consciousness. Do you understand 'You' and 'Outer Mind' are two different entities? The "Inner" is the heart, whilst the "Outer" is the senses and its extension.

The fragrance of a flower, sunset or a dew drop is beautiful. 'MIND' is the most beautiful thing in the World. The mind is endowed with the consciousness itself, and the other end of 'Mind is God'. Mind is a gift from Nature when it is expanded; otherwise it is a pain in the emotional state!

Hence, you have the choice right now to keep enclosed or expand to comprehend the wonders within yourself. The option is to stay in misery, or to remain happily! These are two states of the same being, a state of the emotional well-being as you ponder.

A life-time is wasted, unless you understand the value of the gift of Nature, and the everyday experiences are to uncover the truth. The journey of consciousness is to expand the mind to eternity, and realization of self with the help of a device called "**MIND**".

The emotions, feelings, perceptions and the truth as consciousness, are deep within forming a mini-verse of the varying consciousness. May be a cross section of the mind filled with emotions is the starting point of the study, to unveil the varying emotions submerged in the abyss of the consciousness. It is like a dust clouded over a mirror of pure consciousness.

A little diligence is needed. A little exercise and meditation is required as you reflect, based on the experiences and revelations of truth. It will reveal the truth within the layer of consciousness.

You have to earn the livelihood, don't you? The whole being is alert and aware in challenging situations. A little surprise to the consciousness is required to wake you up. When someone enquired the differences between a common man, and an enlightened; Buddha said: "**You are all sleeping Buddhas** while I am awakened" is the response from Buddha the Enlightened. The views will change; you're in one dimensional view "1D"quality of life, whereas it is a three dimensional view "3D" view in Buddha as they are in a different set of mind in the expanded state.

I read it somewhere in a Zen book.

"Pain is inevitable,

Suffering is optional."

Is it not true? You cannot confront pain; the sufferings can be minimized based on your actions. How often have you realized you are a victim of mind, because of the wrong doing? Perhaps you've realized the importance of mind, and the behavioural analysis.

My opinion is based on the crisis situation; extraordinary circumstances such as an accident, or death of someone near and loved will take you deeper into the heart! This situation will help you transcend conditioning to understand the values within. I am not saying you should deliberate extraordinary circumstances; Indeed, you should be aware of the moments with realization through a psychic process of transformation.

There is no better time to grow in mind; Nature wants you to expand beyond the normal routine in life. The eternal life should not remain confined to survival of the fittest. It should expand and understand everything as the manifestations of Nature. This is called 'LEELA' in Hinduism; infact there is no other purpose in life. The main purpose is to live life to the fullest and appreciate by living in harmony with Nature, and enjoyment of the senses within limits. It has been derailed in between by the social conditioning.

The balance is lost within MIND as you are split. The convictions of truth is lost in hypocrisy. You continue reflecting the surface of 'Mind' as behaviour instead of the root. It is like treating the behaviour of human-conscious which can help to some extent, but it does not help in the realization unless you contemplate it deeply.

There is no magic pill available to extend the spiritual Nature. It needs a particular quality time to spend with inner self. The inner Nature to realize the potential. If you keep on moving in the state of flux, nothing will be certain. You will miss the point always as you have been doing. As you grow biologically, the cumulative past experiences can help you transcend beyond the mundane plane of life. The survival alone is like vegetating with no intentions of living life intensively.

The surface is hankering for the sensual pleasures by spending the energy and the soul passes through the trauma of experiences in births to follow. The Atma (soul) will eventually sublimate karmic influences. It takes centuries to dissipate the karmic influences to merge with the Cosmos. Throughout this or deal, Nature will augment you to achieve the ultimate destiny, which is the ultimate union with the cosmic consciousness. I'll explain each of these points scientifically.

The ultimate choice is to use your media (body) now, or procrastinate it for centuries to achieve the final destination by sublimating your **KARMAS**. If you let the mind wander, it will just gothrough the senses, and fall apart eventually! Perhaps you are hallucinating and living in a hell in this present moment, though it is a real heaven. How would you comprehend the truth, unless you expand your mind?

I read it somewhere '**DROP THE MIND**'. It is not possible to leave the mind until you are dropped dead. Only way is to eliminate the harmful and negative conditioning, and the karmic-debts in mind. Once the mind becomes lighter, it can expand to the super-conscious itself and transform your life to the extraordinary life. Mind is a shadow which should follow the core. You've empowered it so much, you are forcing the core to follow it. Hence the conflict.

The dualities exist in mind because of the conditioning; hence you have to uproot each of them by analyzing; each of its consequences from the subconscious layer of the mind. Unfortunately, it has affected the ability to reach the inner core. The perceptions are based on the MIND, which is the only tool to perceive things. For example, you will be using a microscope to view the cells and virus etc. The ability to perceive things is based on the collective conscious mind which forms the core personality.

Your own interpretations will change if you elevate yourself, by means of meditation and introspective analysis. You are slightly more reactive than being responsive, based on the assumptions; which may not be your realization. It is all based on the past conditioning.

You'll find layers of karmic influences such as desires, temporamental moods that are deep down in the unconscious mind; that are accumulated due to the Genetic imprints. As

59

Bhagvat Gita indicates the types of **KARMAS** known as the 'SANCHITA' karma resulting in reflections of images imprinted deep down. When you intercept each of these; you'll find roots to something else, and it seems to be a never ending reality as you've been gathering **KARMAS** in every event. In addition, there is a bigger baggage that you've accumulated in the 'ACAMIYA' karma, which is the imprints based on your actions till date. The karma, does not necessarily indicate negativity as it could be a 'good' karma, inherited resulting in good virtues in life.

"Is it irony of the truth? Why Nature has provided you with MIND?" It has the capacity to record events and bound by the four factors:

1) Time, 2) Space, 3) Volume and 4) Distance. Mind has the capacity to replay imprints back when needed. The irony is that even GOD cannot go back retroactively in TIME as it is progressive evolution!

Only mind has the capacity to retroactively replay events; with the ability to replay the sensations, thereby causing virtual moods. Nevertheless, virtuous act or immoral act is a different view point. I am just saying the ability to '**RECORD** and **REPLAY**'; if you intend to use mind towards spirituality, it will expand towards the Nature, with the "I" (EGO) disappearing totally!!!

This is not a myth or a Hindu philosophy. It is the fundamental truth in you and me. The secrets of Nature will be revealed to you, when you intercept through constant self-inquiry in silence. GOD loves talking to you, when you aren't talking! You have to raise intellectually, by expanding the ability to receive subtle messages from the cosmic consciousness. I am not talking about the knowledge accumulated in the '**UNIVERSITY**' education. Alright from a commercial perspective for surival, a university degree is required. However, you'll need something beyond as the real education of truth to help you uncover truth.

The cream of Upanishad, Bhagvat Gita in scientific terms relating to the 'GOD' or the 'Unified Force' to demystify all rituals by the way of knowledge and then practices such as Yoga sadhana as realization based curiculam.

The ancient school of wisdom in India taught realization based education known as 'GURUKUL' where students learn from the master's revelations of truth. This is the mode of ancient education taught in the schools of 'Harappa' and 'Mohenjo-daro' of the Indus valley civilization. It had the "Realization based" value system, where you would contemplate to achieve.

The contemporary education has lost all its significance, and it is merely producing mindless robots; These robots are learning basic math and science to acquire some skills with no values in whatsoever in a real life situation. A real education should open the eyes of consciousness, and understand the values of 'CAUSE and EFFECT' system. This is not an instinctive or borrowed knowledge; instead it will be the revelations. Everyone attains biological maturity at the age of twelve, about thirteen or fourteen, and each of you have the capacity to reproduce as per Nature's design. Nature (GOD) wants you to inquire about its creativity,which is the intrinsic quality of mind.

You have so many characters; personalities submerged in the subconscious mind. These are your karmic debts, until and unless cleared at the grass root level, it will always remain as dormant, and emerge once in a while depending on the circumstances. You will never be able to realize it absolutely, and never be able to liaise with the Super conscious; unless your karmic influences are sublimated.

I can only analyze my karmic influences, so as each one of you; I believe Nature (God) has given you the capacity to think, analyze and sublimate each of its consequences. Even so called 'GURU' can't give you any tranquilizer to resolve all problems. They can only give you tools, and methods to analyze!!!

The moods are traces of emotions from the memory; hence it is not real. Instead of tracing the source of every mood and emotions, we keep trying tranquilizers to hold the 'mood' of happiness itself. These moods and emotions will need to be dropped to achieve uninterrupted bliss in mind; if you catch hold of the wrong things, and deeply submerged into the layers of the unconscious mind. Hence, all miseries, anxieties and fear in a day-to-day life as you are going through now.

The sensations are real, and at times these moods are fake ones, and thoughts are in a state of flux, which comes up with consequences of affecting the state of mind. It can either elevate right now or dissipate the energy in negative thinking. The creativity is Natural, and negativity is conditioning, and it is unnatural! The behavioural analysis and diagnosis is required to realize the disorders; however, **identifying** the root is the best. If you would treat the root then, there is no need to chase the state of flux.

Anecdote for you... Treating it at the root.

When a Scientist in Japan was puzzled to find decaying leaves of a plant in a garden in uptown. It seems to be decaying in summer whilst other plants do flourish and flower.

He had conducted various experiments to identify the cause, but all in vain without much of a success in **identifying** the cause! As the Zen master 'DHAMO' arrives in the garden, as he smells the leaves, he found something was different. He investigated the leaves, and veins, where sunlight is pouring; and concludes:

The nutrients to the plant are polluted as the Scientist was not sure.

He said, "son, look at the roots you will find the truth, and he smelled the tip of the roots which was pale."

This is exactly how the behavioural analysis would go. One after the other, the mind is in a constant state of flux. You have symptoms of Alzheimer's disease on day one, when the treatment had started, which turns out to be ADHD disorder hyperactive disorder, so on and so forth. One leading to the other!

The bottom line is that the collective thoughts that are surfacing from the unconscious is the one to treat. You will catch the truth if you are centered within self by way of awareness. All these behaviours have emulated, or conditioned from the animal kingdom which was instinctive, and a need based. Each of these past instincts has reached you in the subconscious state of mind!

Conscious Mind
Sub-conscious/semi-conscious condition
Unconscious Mind

You have several untreated emotions deep down in the subconscious mind, due to conditioning from Genetics through the way of inheritance from your parents, and lineage from the animal behaviour as stated above. These are grouped and indicated in the subconscious state of mind as behavioural patterns. You've empowered negative thoughts; emotions deep down. You seem to be cherishing the harmful effects of it, rather than transforming the way of self-counseling to get away from the conditioning.

A simple analogy, these addictions are somewhere deep down in the subconscious mind, and start emerging from time-to-time as you fuel them. It will excite the required senses, to dissipate the energy (biomagnetism). These negative thoughts will gain prominence, even if you analyze with the conscious mind, at times. The subconscious imprints have been fueled regularly, and ready to erupt at any moment!

Another analogy is like a serpent that looks asleep, but is still awake. This is an excellent example, each of your negative emotion is a serpent that looks like sleeping in the unconscious. It will just sprout up with a '**ssssshhhhhhhhhh**' sound to retaliate you at any moment.

A little awareness will help you get over the condition. The conditioning in the collective subconsciousness will need analysis, by witnessing. The personalities are not fixed entities. This is exactly the reason why saints become sinners, or perhaps the other way. It all happens, depending on what is there being the semi and subconscious mind.

The personality traits varies based on the environment, social, and the behaviour changes depending on the baseline assumptions. Hence, it is required to have a reason based culture, and knowledge to sharpen the intellect; in order to practice awareness, which should become your intrinsic quality. Otherwise, you would repeat things in a cyclic pattern and repent, and feel guilty forever. Nature has endowed with the ability to think, analyze, visualize and realize.

These facets of mind can help you heal yourself by way of expanding it to the super-consciousness. You cannot treat behavioural disorders such as ODD or ADHD (hyperactive) or Schizophrenic conditions through medications. Only way is to identify the root causes of trauma in childhood or Genetics, and recondition it to grow positively in spiritual aspects. Otherwise, medications won't help much to alleviate pains from the current situation. It is just restricted to treating the parts of the physiology, and not treated at psychology!

This will give you some temporary relief but not a solution to the impending problems in life. It would further complicate as your neurons are weakened, and apparently you would end up losing the ability to think effectively. This will result in a different disorder which your medical journal will name it as another disorder.

Do not catch the behaviour, only identifying the root is beneficial. Instead of saying "my mind is thinking" about 'this', and negatively, try to rephrase it by saying: "my mind is Contemplating about itself". **Who am I? What is my origin?** When you develop the inner inquisitiveness to look inward, to examine at self, and the behaviour.

This behavioural pattern will change. GOD will help you when you seek advice! It is a basic law of Nature! When you are thinking about a beautiful morning sunshine, what happens to your mind? You will become the 'object' itself, which is a 'sunshine' as the mind takes the form. A beautiful place in mind is a beautiful projection stored such as liaising with Nature. It is played back as a sensation, whenever you want to retrieve. It depends on what you want in life, streaming blissful life or miseries to continue through the life! Perhaps you have been conditioned to feel depressed without being aware of it. This feeling would ruin you at any moment.

The mind hallucinates and creates one hundred and one things without any rationale! There is no ghost out there, except for the ghosts within each of you! The deadliest mind could be none other than your mind if not harnessed properly. There is no other way to realize GOD without analyzing the tool called '**Mind**'.

Are you aware of all that is happening beyond the senses? It is a labyrinthine going within yourself in physics, chemistry and biology; at all layers of physical and mental plane which you are constantly ignoring. Since, you are endowed with the most beautiful mind; you are not recognizing its importance.

Would you work for achieving something that you do not have now? You have a desire to buy a beautiful home and car or bike! Did you ever think about the beautiful mind; the eternal home perceiving everything, and replaying? It is not just a response from the brain; there is a little more electromagnetic discharge through the brain cells as responses called "**THINKING**".

Perceptions

Perceptions

Conditioning

The perceptions are based on the 'baseline' conditioning as you evaluate each situation based on what you have accumulated. What I have observed is so many wrong conditioning; resulting in addictions. You can only get out of addictions by changing your perceptions.

Can sensory perceptions alone bring you happiness? You keep thinking, analyzing as though money, sex and power are the only things that will give you pleasure. The lust for money or power is based on the social setup with false sensations. The real intent should be helping you attain your real self.

I'll teach you "AVR" method to help you get over the conditioning.

The "AVR" ("Analyze-Visualize-Realize") Method.

Perhaps you should try and change the baseline condition with intelligence, which is the real analysis based on your revelations.

Perceive through intelligence

Intelligence out of consciousness; and you would be aware of the situation eventually.

Let us analyze the originating thoughts where are they coming from?

Thoughts and Actions

The perceptions will change based on the cumulative experiences. By realizing pains from the past doing and the effects. It is the right time to improve the perceptions, and segregate what is the cause of your pain and analyze. Just become more aware of the present moments, by dropping the past wrong doing which you are holding.

Whatever you gain as knowledge will let you react, unless you are acting based on your own revelations of truth. Hence, it will need extra effort to analyze the behaviour using mind mapping techniques. Identify the source of all problems, analyze each of these situations and understand the cause.

Formula: "thoughts-actions-results"

The harmful results can be eliminated by filtering the thoughts and actions. Hence, you should be aware of every single thought. These thoughts can either propel you towards extreme '**OUTER**' through the senses or '**INNER**' aligned to the consciousness.

Thoughts are extremely powerful, and it has manifested in to actions based on thinking, and eventually it becomes your character. The results are also manifestations of thoughts. If you are leading a miserable life, just stop the routine activities for a week or two, think about every single thought and ways to transcend it by intellectual inquiry.

At the most, you would condemn 'failures' with some excuses, and you'll find a way to escape by consuming alcohol, which is a lot easier than contemplation or meditation. This is a perfect recipe to start the engine and let go with closed eyes. Mind will remain closed when you're drunk! The dreams are projections of the subconscious mind. It looks so real! You seem to be addicted to the sensations and a dream of happiness, not the alcohol.

When you are drunk, the whole world seems to be listening to you and everything happens in accord. The next day is even more painful as the hangover is gone! When the beautiful dreams stop, or if you realize it is a dream you will hanker for the reality. The reality is within you, deep within layers of your consciousness awaiting your return. Have you observed every emotion has a boundary? The recharge mechanism is provided to you as a gift as 'sleep' by Nature. It recharges your batteries while you are asleep, and then you are ready to move in the morning.

"Have you observed who is healing in the interim, and how much do you owe?" Don't you pay the one, who has repaired your Porche parked right there! And the regular maintenance at a free of charge. This is exactly what Nature has endowed you with at no expense. First, you have the ability to enjoy sensations by expanding your own energy within moderation. It is perceived by mind as pleasure.

'What is causing these sensations and who is feeling happy or sad?' A brief realization of the above facets of your emotions, sensations and moods can heal you! The past conditioning is extremely easy to eliminate. The irony is that, the moment you think of anything, mind will assume the shape of the object, and depending on the wavelength you subject it to...the consequences will be beneficial or awful. It can turnout either positive, or negative, depending on what you had invited!

My own observation is that God never intended to give you anything **"negative"**. It is all experiences. If you do not oblige to the **"Laws of Nature"**, and **"CAUSE and EFFECT"** theory you go over the board, and spend the energy to a large extent. Thus, resulting in misaligned cellular structure, causing unpleasant sensations called 'pain' as a result of your action, there is nothing else. Nature has manifested itself as results. It's all energy phenomenon!

You are clear with the conditioning. Now, a radical change is required; After having understood the facets, with the realization of the ultimate Laws of Nature. It is you, who is spending the inner energy, which results in pain or pleasure. **"Whom else to be blamed?"** None other than yourself!

If you are going through an experience of trauma, it could be due to past conditioning, and the repetitive pattern in terms of addiction to the senses causing neurological disorders. You may call it as Schizophrenic, or Alzheimer or **ADHD** or **ODD**.

These are the entire behavioural pattern due to some cause! I would like you to analyze the cause of the conditioning due to karmic influences. The only way is to introspective analysis to change the roots to change behaviour, consequently the personality itself. I believe there is no short-cut to propose medications to resolve this.

A profound technique is to remain being silent for 1 hour a week, and gradually increase it to a few hours/week; if you practice being silent with no or limited thoughts in mind, then you will be centered to the consciousness; you will find a conditioning emerging one after the other, from the subconscious mind?

Otherwise, you would fall as a victim to the emerging situation, due to the trauma experiences of the past conditioning passing by, if you are not determined, then you will subject the whole being suffering in sensations of 'pain', and the present moments are lost. In ancient Hinduism, saints called it as '**Thirikal Naan**' meaning intelligence to analyze the past events, evaluate the current circumstances, and estimate the future results. You have the capacity to do it.

A disciple asked Buddha about the future events:

Oh master! "**How is it possible to realize all future events manifesting?**"

Buddha smiled at him and said:

"The Enlightened master is the one who remains in unison with Nature and whatever he thinks is in unison with Nature. The following events are the manifestations of current circumstances, where I am just living in the moment to moment awareness."

Ok. Let's discuss the artifacts of ignorance or innocence which are different state of minds. Either you choose to be ignorant, or act innocent; hence the sufferings in your life.

Ignorance Vs. Innocence

As we discussed mind conditioning; perhaps you can explain the origin of conditioning, or even the behavioural analysis to children at an early age. When a boy or girl reaches 14-15 years of age, the sexual energy is at its prime. The intelligence levels are dependent on how you harness the energy towards higher values as you grow, assuming you have experienced enough in life to comprehend values of truth. This would help in visualizing past instances, to help you transcend from all types of conditioning. The realization of truth should become your inherent quality.

The children are Innocent, like simple mirrors, reflecting the imprints. The possible ways to change their conditioning is by way of inculcating habits and techniques of lowering their mental frequency, and simple fables that would help them succeed. This would help them in handling the situations at an adult stage.

If you are ignorant as an adult, then there is no excuse, rather by the law of '**CAUSE** and **EFFECT**', you will experience the consequences as pain. Eventually you would learn; but how do you learn is extremely beneficial. If you can understand it intellectually; and understand that fire is a danger, and be caution while using it. You will automatically refrain from it. If you do not realize the effects of your own doing, may be you will end up realizing at last, when most part of your life is gone already!

You do not need '**STD**' type of sexual diseases and/or hypertension, cardiovascular or neurological disorders in mind revealing your past instances. You have not taken enough time to ponder on yourself! Nature is the result. And the cause is your '**Action**', and the result is God as '**Reaction**'. A paradigm shift is required in you realizing GOD as manifestations, force and as "**everlasting, singular, and mighty divine fluid.**"

A simple analogy; If you clap your hands, it will create a sound. There is a conversion of pressure into sound, which is 'GOD's effect, and the 'CAUSE' is 'CLAPPING', isn't it?

Mind has been gifted to you by Nature to realize the eternity in self, and not intended for sensory perceptions alone. As stated earlier visualize the impact without being subjected to the emotions. The outer mind will record what you think and do precisely, and it will provoke the subconscious mind. Eventually, the conscious mind will succeed if practiced diligently into various compelling circumstances. There is no need to go to Himalayas for silence. The challenge is to succeed in the market place. Be in the world, and transcend after experiencing through every situation in life.

"Martin and Krish meet at a nearby Tai restaurant in the downtown for the next session."

"Krish orders for a fish and sausage with chips, along with a Tai made wine. It's authentic."

Let's try these first:

"Here is the appetizer. The chinese dragon wings and open the small piece of paper, which is your fortune for the day!!!"

Martin was very excited as he opens it up.

"Be a light unto you."

Martin looks at Krish thinking, this could be his plan. "Don't look at me Martin," this is your fortune. A real fortune to realize.

Let me explain:

"You'll need to be aware as ZEN portrays in every moment-to-moment awareness. Just watch out!" Krish is pointing out to the ceiling with a hanging naked sword!!!!

"Oh no. The moments changed." Martin was suddenly awake and joy transformed into alertness.

"What are you thinking, Mr. Martin?" The situation turned a little intense. Krish pointed him to calm down, and be seated and enjoy the food.

"What am I thinking? Damn it. I am not thinking anything." he jumped out of the sword that was hanging in there above his head.

"Is that a trick?" he asked Krish.

"Yes, that is!!! This is not a real sword! Nevertheless, how did you feel?"

"I felt nervous, and then alert to protect my life from being killed by a naked sword. Were you thinking about food?"

"Initially yes, but when I saw my life was in danger I was alert!!! I was thinking about the danger above my head."

"This is a natural response, no conditioning perhaps," Krish chuckles.

"Didn't you realize being Aware?"

"Of course, yes, for few moments. There is no better way having learnt this exercise," he chuckles.

Both leave for the rest of the evening. Martin contemplates on the instances of significance which is a life changing game as he thought to himself!!!

You can practice the above technique to get over the conditioning, and also succeed in transcending from senses based semi-conscious to the conscious Mind. Being alert, and conscious about instances instead of being influenced by conditioning. Replacing it with alert and conscious thinking. It will be your revelations of truth which will guide you.

Martin, you know about these sensations-beyond sensations and enjoyment in moderation.We talked about conditioning; my next session will be in **identifying** the roots of conditioning, which is MIND. See you there next week! Dr. drives away in his Porsche.

"Thanks Dr.!" Martin walks out with regained confidence.

You've mastered the first four rules of The 7 Golden Rules of Zen Wisdom:

> **Identify 'SENSATIONS' (IYS);**
>
> **Look 'BEYOND' the Sensations (LBS);**
>
> **Enjoyment in 'MODERATION' (EM);**
>
> **Know Your 'CONDITIONING' (KYC).**

In the next session, we will analyze the social conditioning and addictions briefly, Martin walks away eagerly awaiting for the next session.

End of Session # 6

3
Social Conditioning

Day 6 – Session # 7:

Today, I am going to teach you about the conditioning of MIND.

Let me start off with an anecdote.

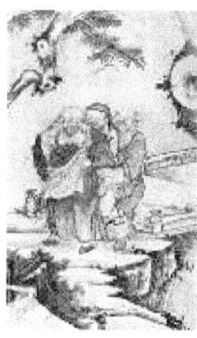 Sometimes you feel happy, and at times you are unhappy for no reason at all. Is there any rationale to the emotions, mood swings? It is like a wild pendulum swaying. Perhaps you will need to check out the old pendulum clock which is truly fascinating. This is an antique piece in the contemporary world of Electronics. It is good to observe a pendulum swaying on either side, which is synonymous to the emotions.

There is something which you have not understood, perhaps the moods, a little closer inspection would yield resulting in emotions, which comes out of the subconsciousness mind. Thereby you realize it as a 'positive' or 'negative' emotions!

You keep holding on to the emotional thread indicated below, let us analyze the facts of your mood swings;

Strings Of Emotions

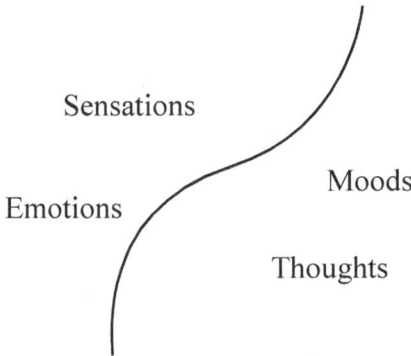

Sensations

Emotions

Moods

Thoughts

Can you write down the mood that you are in now, and the emotional feelings that you are going through in the moment while you are reading this book? I have another example from a Psychiatrist as indicated below from a patient's record; "I feel resentment in myself right now and guilty at times, sad and depressed and at times passionate about sex and so forth."

"I am feeling "GUILTY", resentment." I've analyzed these findings in one of the workshops based on inputs from the participants; A Zen technique to eliminate negative emotions. Let us analyze each of these emotions. Perhaps the mood swings are caused by these emotions; as you move further closer to the moods.

It would result in sensations of either pain, or pleasure. Perhaps "Peaceful" state, which is a neutral position of mind, you might be astonished to find the other side of pleasure is pain; This corollary helps. It has a profound meaning as you may think the pain is far off. The pain is always much closer, as much as you feel happy right now. The sensations of peace are a non-linear function in your mind. As it takes a lot of practice to stabilize, and remain in the neutral state.

"I am feeling 'ANGRY'". You feel anger right now, someone wanted to kill someone else. I have heard in a workshop! Why is it so? It is deep down in the subconscious mind; these imprints remain untreated for years. you have been carrying so many imprints known as the past "**KARMAS**".

These **KARMAS** are inherited from the single sense plant to the sixth sense, through the evolutionary process of Genetics. When each of these emotions is untreated, it will stimulate instinctive behaviour from the subconscious mind. A simple analogy of anger repressed temporarily would result in extreme rage, and it will erupt like a volcano, awaiting its turn! Anyone who claims to be good, the so called "Religious" entities have been suppressing emotions for a while, and they are the foremost ones to watch out!

A real situation will evoke such emotions, changing the character to harm others. Perhaps an emotion can start as a need based such as "hunger". The survival of the fittest, as Darwin says in the animal kingdom; It is instinctive in the animals. If the basic-needs are not fulfilled, there will be a strong desire to sublimate. This is quite Natural!

The human endeavour of consciousness is to purify **KARMAS** and to realize the Divine Nature. I strongly believe this is the purpose of life. Often, I have realized this expansion of mind will give you absolute peace. This is the neutral state of mind with fewer emotions as you grow spiritually.

Hence, it is your responsibility to realize the creativity of the Divine Nature, by observing each of these emotions, mood swings and transcend through intellectual reasoning. The mind will require additional inputs to convert animal instincts; through introspective analysis that will help you transcend emotions into an elevated state of consciousness.

The entire body is subjected to the emotional state of mind in a state of excitement; resulting in its own consequences. The irony is that when you remain enclosed in an emotion, your whole being is in a state of flux. For example, if you're angry, your rate of the blood stream flow increases, and heartbeat increases. The body temperature increases, which is unnatural, resulting in chaos with the human physiology and psychology.

When I analyze your responses, it is predominantly an excited state of mind causing disturbances to your neurons, brain cells and the body cells. Perhaps the most emotional unstable people, are the ones who are prone to heart diseases? It is due to rapid changes to the blood circulation which is not streamlined due to improper emotional imbalance.

You have to become emotionally stable. And there are basic needs that you will need to fulfil, such as **food, rest, sex** and **work**. Each of it should be in moderation in order to stabilize your emotions. Any depressions will cause adverse consequences in any of the four facts discussed above. Well. Let me ask you this. Are you a victim of these sensations or the observer? Often you are a victim!!! Perhaps you've not analyzed enough to get closer within yourself to identify the discreet truths, which are lying dormant in you.

Have you noticed if you think about the past trauma experiences, your consciousness will open up? An experience closer to the heart, where the above analogy would reveal facts of your mood swings, sensations, and emotions. Seldom, you did analyze it within yourself. The thread of emotions can cause sensations of pain or pleasure. The pain is nothing but a form of disarrays in the biological function, and emotions are a result of a transformation of the energy.

Why is there a constant conflict in your analysis? You tend to perform a task in a specific mental wavelength; and then repent for the wrong doing as a guilt consciousness. The reason is that due to the past conditioning. The prefix notation in your mind is set with incorrect calculations. A simple analogy of maths would prove as no one can deny:

"(a+b)2=a2+b2+2ab...(1)". If you are assuming it as "(a+b)2=a2+b2......(2)"; then your basics aren't right?

Now, you would comprehend by saying it is my incorrect calculations after you realize. This is exactly what is happening in your life as you miscalculate everything without aligning with the "**Laws of Nature**". As per the "**CAUSE and EFFECT**" theory, Nature is precise calculations as it would yield as results, based on your actions. Now, you tell me whose responsibility is this?

Who is responsible for all your sufferings? It's none other than "YOU". You have chosen the path of the arduous journey, denying the truth.

For example, you say 'I studied Engineering; however, I desire to be the best Doctor in the World at some point after seeing many Doctors around'. Just observe the rationale behind your desires. There is no rationale in anything. You assume being happy, only after achieving the goal of '$ X' USD Million. In reality, once you achieve 'X' million, you're sad than before! I believe happiness is a state of mind that you'll need to practice.

'You were dating a beautiful woman, and your relationships have failed many times'. What happens next, after you marriage, your happiness ends after a couple of years? If your love is eternal, may be you should feel the same way till the end right. Perhaps your mind is in a state of flux, which is desiring for above and beyond the mundane plane of life. This is absolutely Natural, and your mind cannot be satisfied unless you attach it with the Eternity. The Natural law is to let the river reach the ocean. If it is stagnated, it is wasted. This is exactly, what is happening in you. You get stagnated without moving on towards eternity.

The mind is in a constant state of flux, as everything changes with the perceptions. The most beautiful woman whom you are in love with at one point changes, not that the woman changes! It is the notion of beauty in you changes! You tend to perceive things differently based on the prefixed notion. Is there anyone guiding you to think about these "notions" to align with the universal laws of truth?

Is this a valid assumption of desiring for something not possible? This is how you have accumulated every thought of cumulative desires without any rationale, thus claiming it "1+1=3".

The above conditioning in mind with an incorrect analysis could result in different emotional state of Mind. Your emotional well-being is the primary importance point above anything in the WORLD.

Rule # 4: Know Your Conditioning (KYC) addictions and Get over

"It's been a life changing experience Dr." Martin is overwhelmed with the analysis of the Dr.

"True, if you'd practice it."

"Ok. Let's do this today."

"Let's draw the artifacts of the conditioning."

"You should start at the centre by writing down the conditioning one-by-one that you may want to get rid. Put down all the negative conditioning. I would draw something much simpler and easy to follow, unlike the above picture."

Your Fluctuating Moods

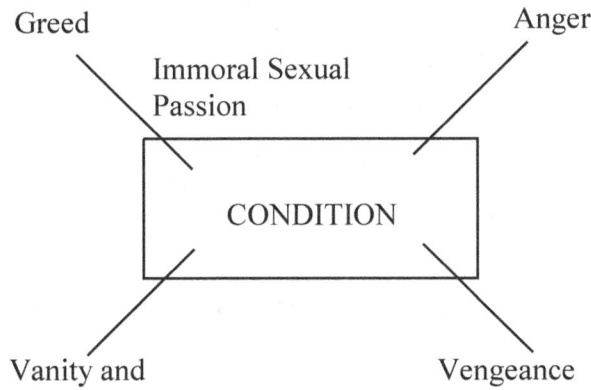

"Martin started filling the boxes in the chart."

"Good Job! Martin. A lot of it to analyze. Ok. You see the centre box indicates your baseline conditioning and the emotions circumventing it, as a result of your conditioning. Let's pick one for the session today. Your immoral sexual passion."

"Why do you call it immoral?"

"Dr. Perhaps it isn't real."

"You mean to say it is virtual, a mind thing."

"Of course Dr."

"Ok. Your perception is carrying on to the virtual sensations and not real. In other words it is a false sensation."

"Yes."

"Now, you have realized it is not a bodily urge at times."

"Yes. Habits."

"I would call it conditioning."

"Ok. Dr."

"Catch the roots of sensations."

"Yes, it is due to the subconscious mind hankering for it."

"We talked about it. It is surfacing out from the subconscious mind. What was a need based as TRUE sensation has turned to FALSE sensations as addictions."

"Hence, you hanker for the sensations."

Ummmmmm… he breaths in deeply with a sigh of relief.

"Now, you change the perceptions."

"Go beyond the sensations."

"ASK YOURSELF. Is this a REAL or FALSE sensations?"

"It isn't real!!!!"

"Keep going, analyze its conditioning."

"Yes Dr." You were made to believe those girls are beautiful. Ask yourself, what is a real beauty."

"Body is beautiful."

"Yes, indeed, a little more….her curves.

"Ok. Good," then...

"Breasts."

Dr. interrupts...

"Well. Can you think beyond the body?"

"Her heart, loving heart and beautiful eyes."

Hmmmm. that's poetic. Beautiful. First one is good, and the second one is better and the third one is the best.

"What is the third one Dr.?"

"**Consciousness or ATMA (micro consciousness)**" which is the eternal beyond Body, and Mind. The centre of **MIND** is consciousness itself. This is the most precious thing in the World.

"Thanks Dr.!" Martin walks out of the session with a deep sigh of relief!!!

End of Session # 7

Dr. Richard is looking at a picture with Swami ji and he thinks about his past life changing experiences in the foothills of Himalyas.
(1955-2030)

Dr. Richard's childhood:

Dr. Richard's father was addicted to drinking, and at a later stage died due to the sexually transmitted diseases, which had left an inundated mark in his mind to analyze the root cause all miseries.

Dr. Richard was the best student in school. He was very good in science, and a brilliant student as his teachers admired

81

him. He went to medical school in South Carolina. There, he became involved in research under the direction of a physiology professor named Ernst. Ernst could not answer all his queries. Dr. Richard had spent many years in analyzing personality to neurology.

Dr. Richard was very good at his research, concentrating on neurophysiology, even inventing a special cell-staining technique. But only a limited number of positions were available, and there were others ahead of him. Ernst helped him to get a grant to study, first with the great psychiatrist Dr. Schultz in Wisconsin. Both these gentlemen were investigating the use of hypnosis with hysterics.

After spending a short time as a resident in neurology and director of a children's ward in Miami, he came back to South Carolina, married his fiancée of many years Emily, and set up a practice in neuropsychiatry with the help of Richard's books and lectures which brought him both fame and from the mainstream of the medical community. He drew around him a number of very bright sympathizers who became the core of the psychoanalytic movement in South Carolina.

Dr. Richard was thinking about his past instances during the college days, and his travel across the world in quest for truth and happiness.

"I've changed my perceptions after my long tour to the hills of Himalayas and my intimate dialogue within myself; neither Mind nor its conditioning is terrible. Perhaps, God is smart enough to endow us with "MIND", with a vow of helping the younger generations, to realize the magnanimous consciousness; In addition the evolution of consciousness with conditioning is a challenge to reckon."

His memories were around the foot hills of Himalayas where he meets a Sadhu.

"Maharishi, What is the root cause of all sufferings in life?"

"My son, these sufferings are due to your past **KARMAS** and lack of knowledge in analyzing **CAUSE and EFFECT** system."

"You continue to act as per the **KARMAS**, though you have the ability to analyze and transcend."

"Why is it so?"

"Because, you need understanding of the laws of Nature and "Willpower" to change the past. You'll be able to achieve only through the Yoga sadhana!"

"Thank You Maharishi!"

He learns unique techniques to relate to the senses. This instance transforms his life, he then practices meditation and spends few months in the hills of Himalayas in silence. These sufferings are due to the karmic influences, which is "CONDITIONING" in the journal of Psychiatry. Well. If these are the excited pattern of imprints and the research takes him to a different plane of mind to formulate '7 Golden Rules of Zen Wisdom' as the unique therapy techinques to help millions of people.

His inner voice tells him:

YOU'RE BORN TO WIN,

BUT CONDITIONED TO FAIL,

THE SUCCESS IS WITHIN YOU,

THROUGH THE INTELLECT,

"GO TEACH THE WORLD."

These words echoing from deep within his heart, he walks with a conviction to formulate workshops that would heal the conditioning of millions to help them getting out of addictions.

Dr. Richard finds his answers in silence.

"Eureka". I'll teach the world as he starts from the hills of Himalayas to the United States. A new journey has just begun!!!

Life is just a passage of learning in the journey of consciousness towards eternity.

Dr. Richard prepared himself for the next session.

Day 7 – Session # 8:
Learn Avr Method

This is a formidable challenge to speak the truth in honest revelations as you would have ignored if you had it with no efforts; hence, God has created an"LEELA" or a play as you call it to go through the situations, analyze, replay and correct it through mind and become aware. Otherwise, Life would be on the rocks with no learning. There is a reason to everything in God's manifestations.

The nearer you get to the two-dimensional (2D) view of the consciousness; your approach will change, and every event will yield the truth. Perhaps you would find life as mysterious, blissful as everlife would be an ecstatic endeavour. The society is one of the reasons for conditioning, and the universities, education has conditioned the mind. The real virtues can come only within you by the revelations, and not by accumulating knowledge. Unfortunately, religions have failed to create virtues.

IDEALISM

REVELATIONS/VIRTUES

CONDITIONING

Only Science will prevail in the future generations, and the conditioning will get stronger, due to the lack of the holistic realization of truth. The practices of meditation and yoga will help you regain the lost consciousness, and introspection will provide you the "**IDEALISM**" to form the baseline conditioning.

How do you evaluate 'right' or 'wrong' or perhaps the virtues that a religion teaches you. When you evaluate through "**The principles of Virtues**" is based on the inner revelation, it becomes clear, and there is no need to force it upon you. For example, Every religion claims its own GOD as the main GOD. Perhaps a little revelation would help you understand 'GOD is one and the same', and the scientific research in Einstein's theory of relativity would help you comprehend the truth as 'mechanics of force'., The static and the dynamic. The '**YIN**' and '**YAN**' as indicated in the chinese philosophy. If you validate based on these scientific revelations, the outcome would be different. There is a difference in a Pilot flying a plane Vs. a Driver driving a car. They both are driving a vehicle, but they are different in terms of analyzing it based on the intellectual reasoning. This is true, when it comes to life. If you live a life at the surface, you will not be able to transcend anything. You will need to raise the quest against everything to identify through the inner revelations.

It becomes a Natural process to validate and accept upon. In a way, it is beneficial to study the behavioural science and link it to the root causes of one of the six temperamental moods as highlighted. It would help you to identify the past conditioning a little deeper. You will be totally aware to realize what you have earned; when you are filled in with the energy.

Let's say some day you become a '**MILLIONAIRE**'; through hard work and dedication, realizing the pain of earning. You will certainly plan for the savings in the bank-account. In a similar way, meditation is beneficial to restore the energy. If it is not streamlined, energy accumulated will be wasted. This should be governed properly like an expense account with reasons of spending through the senses. You will soon become void of it and the balance would yield nil.

You might have heard about a great saint. "**Vishwamitra**", who is a kshatriya a community of Kings by birth, hence he was easily resorted to anger, and moods of passion when he was seduced. He had these elements of past conditioning. Eventually he got tricked by a Gandharva, (heavenly women) to check his convictions of truth; he succumbs to passion, and anger. This is perhaps a real story, unless you counsel each of your conditioning, it is just a matter of time and the opportunity presenting itself. Each of these opportunities is a manifestation of your thoughts. The past dreams are fueled by the mind-power, by replaying the instances, which would influence your subsequent actions, resulting in positive or negative results.

These passions will be multifold, and anger will be hurting deeper. The imprints are there in the genetics, taking you far away from the spirituality. Hence, you will need to comprehend the behaviour based on the past conditioning, realize the core personality. This will need a little counseling within self even before you start practices of meditation and introspection. Once you learn basic and simple techniques of breathing and meditation; you should combine meditation and introspective analysis.

Each of this conditioning is linked to the subconscious mind; you should plan to dissipate it righteously by analysis or sublimate negative emotions by superimposing with a positive emotion. For example, If you are addicted to alcohol or smoking; your lungs are spoiled and Dr. has advised you to refrain from! Now, you realize the harmful behaviour and you plan to stop it. You have to recondition your mind by way of using mind power to empower positive thoughts. Remember, I am not saying '**Control thoughts'**; instead, empower the positive thoughts. The negativity will sublimate by itself. The only way you can do it is by meditation. You will gain positive mind power and empower the positive thoughts, for a win-win situation.'

A few years ago, there was a witchcraft lady in her early thirties, in the voodoo lounge sought my help to treat her patient.

"Dr. Richard, could you please help me?"

"Yes. What is the matter, Hana?"

"I am going to tell you about Nancy."

When I enquired her in my session to find the spirit. She was totally possessed by a spirit which didn't want to leave her body.

I asked the spirit, which claimed to be over a FIVE HUNDRED YEARS OLD, and she wanted to revenge a King, Solomon IV.

"Interesting." Dr. was looking more inquisitively.

I have examined her. "The spirit is looking forward to revenging a King, who had killed her in the past life!!! After centuries, there was no Kingdom. But the spirit wanted to revenge him."

"True. These spirits are not bound by TIME. Dr. Richard charts out a game plan to help Hana."

"Ok. Let's do this. And treat her psychology of soul."

"What do you mean Dr.?"

"I mean treating a spirit's psychology. The spirit has been conditioned, which need to be resolved through Psychiatry."

"Ok. Let's meet next weekend. He had prepared a studio with casts of a King, with few soldiers etc. It looked like a Hollywood cast with required palace to stage the show."

Dr. Richard cast himself as King Solomon. He looked like a King Solomon IV.

"That's impressive," she claimed.

The whole drama was formed to trick the evil spirit by creating an illusion, and an act of stage drama to help it cures the imprint psychologically, by satisfying the spirit.

The evil spirit in her body, yelled "Kill the damn bastard, he had raped and killed me."

She came forward on the stage, and the warrior helps him with a sword to cut King Solomon's head, which is the dummy head.

The dummy head rolls off to the ground!!! The SPRIT, cherished every moment of the revenge taken against the king.

The dummy body was lying down. Dr. Richard was taken underneath the stage to another place. The entire play was made to treat the psychology of the spirit in order to remove its past conditioning.

Hana thanks to Dr. Richard for all his help!

"Martin, I am going to teach you my research outcome, AVR method."

"What is the AVR method Dr.?"

"It indicates Analyze-Visualize-Realize."

It is based on my research, each of your conditioning is a deep wound of the past and trials of past events in sequences. It is endowed with the circles of convoluted theories around with two sets of arguments of 'right' and 'wrong'. The 'virtues' and 'sins'; and neither of them are strong enough to win the battle.

It seems like a constant battle between the 'Bad Guys' Vs. 'Good Guys' within each of you. Eventually, the 'bad-guys' win as they are always stronger as you infuse more negativity through the mind-power. It is like using a nuclear reactor to generate electricity or using it to destroy a country! The mind-power should be used constructively.

In the deepest split, known as schizophrenic split in minds and the conditioning. It emerges from the unconscious to the conscious. Hence, you feel painful, and most of you take tranquilizers with sleeping pills. There is no way to get closer to the heart as you are hooked up to the gadgets almost 24X7. Then, how can you expect peace as you are not allowing peace to enter in the heart with the wired gadgets. Your mind becomes a chatter box.

Perhaps Nature will reflect your conditioning as the centre is associated with the Universal centre and it is interlinked. It is always everlasting, which would help in a crisis situation with all solutions to your problems coming from within. All problems exist due to the conditioned mind at the surface, whereas the solution exists at the centre of the core consciousness. Everything is interconnnected as the saying goes 'You cannot pluck a flower without disturbing a distant planet.'

Unfortunately, you look for the resolution everywhere except within yourself. When you are centered, the answers will come from within, with an attunement of self in a specific wavelength. The frequency of Mind is measured in Cycles per Second (CPS) with the 'Electro Encephala Gram'; which is a device used for measurement of mental frequency. Perhaps the EEG tells you whether you are happy or sad or whatever as each of these sensations causes a specific sensation in a particular wavelength.

Do you know that mind is wave, and the mental wavelength is measured in frequency? Don't you realize the moods depend on the mental wavelength? Beta is 14-40CPS, Alpha-7-17 CPS. Theta is 3-6 and finally Delta is the subtlest state of Mind 1-3. Perhaps if you are able to achieve Delta state of mind for even a split second. One dimensional (1D) view of mind changes to three dimensions in everything you do. The endeavour of consciousness will continue.

Often, when I tried to practice silence, these imprints will play the spoil sport which remains as untreated emotions deep in the subconscious mind. When it surfaces, it will dust the conscious mind and impair the senses. More so, senses do have particular imprints, which may take over the consciousness mind. It is like a robotic arm engaging controlling rather than brain controlling through neurons. For example, if you are addicted to food; even when your mind says it as wrong, you will go-ahead with overeating. Have you observed? You were instructed by the mind, but the senses have taken control. This is exactly what I mean by senses going out of sync due to addictions. This applies to all senses.

If you catch the behavioural pattern, you'll be able to identify sensations, and the cause being one of the six temperamental moods as stated. The only way is to address the roots, not the leaves.

How would you validate an event in Mind? It is through the experience, and the sensations are the part of your mind, which evaluates a specific event. The irony is that what you may consider as beauty, wonder is perhaps not rely in the exact state. For the instance, What you may perceive as beauty is just a one dimensional (1D) view due to your short-sight and conditioning. Perhaps there is a larger connotation to the beauty itself. If you examine this closely through the intellectual reasoning and self-inquiry, you will understand the beauty as the Nature itself. It is not in the object, it is certainly in the subject in mind and inner perceptions.

As we discussed, Mind assumes the shape or volume of any object that you perceive, hence the real beauty lay in the perceptions based on the past conditioning. What I am saying is that Jack may assume a beauty differently than Jill. It all depends on the individual characterization and personality whilst someone may find it different.

The core of the mind is the consciousness itself. You will find a third dimensional (3D) view which is a paradigm shift in everything, and you will laugh at the primal conditions and the animal instincts; as you have the ability to reflect on every single event from your childhood till now as an adult, to reflect, analyze, visualize and realize. In order to get to this understanding, you will need to "stand-under", which means a subtle state of mind attuned to realize the facts in discreet terms.

Analyze

|

Visualize

|

Realize

The above three qualities of analysis can yield success in getting over the past conditioning by intensive form of introspective analysis and meditation. You have the ability to be responsive, instead of being reactive in every situation. For example, you can choose to be angry, or without anger to find a resolution plan. Every situation should go through analysis in mind, visualizing the impact of it and the realization of result. You do not need to burn the fingers to realize 'fire' should be used carefully. You will know the results upfront like visualizing the awareness of 'fire' and realize the outcome, as stated in the above analysis.

The choice is to be passionate right now and analyze if it is needed based real of fake emotions. It is all within you, and no one can perhaps look at what is going on in your mind. Each of you is a multiverse, made up of Pancha-boothas, the five elements: **Land, Water, Fire, Air and Energy particles**. The irony is that you have not been educated to realize your greatness, instead taught to be as brave as '**Alexander, who is termed to be the great'**. Perhaps the great who has killed so many people in the name of war. The greatness is in the power of the mind, and the realization like a Buddha to emulate! Whereas history has taught you the power of muscles in the name of '**ALEXANDER THE GREAT'**.

"In summary, you have to analyse a specific situation, visualize the outcome and realize the benefit. If it yields good, then support it. You have to be aware in every moment by practicing A-V-R method, before you are surprised by sequences of events."

Relationships

Martin,

You've had problems with the relationships right. Do you know the reason why all relationships are on rocks? The reason is that you fail to recognize the value of it; resulting in the negative consequences. You were ignorant of the Law of Nature. Did you analyze the relationships, and why most of the marriages are on the rocks?

There is a reason for everything as per the Nature's design. These imprints (karmic-debts) are attracting the spouse based on the sixteen pattern of imprints. God wanted you to sublimate the karmic influences, through the spouse and progress in the journey of consciousness. It is like a mug needs a lid to close it and a circuit will need to close.

In Hindu mythology, The male energy and female energy have to complete by forming a closed circuit. This is the significance of Lord. SIVA in 'ARDHANARI' which means, half-man and half-woman, which depicts the complete cycle.

Your mind is half-male and half-female; hence, you will need a spouse to share the imprints to sublimate over a period of time. This is a gracefulness of the Divine Nature. First it had created you through the evolutionary process, and then he wanted you to drop the conditioning by realizing it. Finally, sublimate all karmic influences by expanding the mind to the consciousness. The life partner will help you in this journey as per Nature's design. Since, you were not in the expanded state of mind, you have constantly missed the point.

Somewhere you seem to get stuck. The reason is that you have not realized the inner values. How would you realize the value of the spouse? Hence, women are ill-treated anywhere in the World, regardless of the culture and the evolution.

"It is a shame that women are just treated as the sexual entities, and it showcases the education, universities which have failed to inculcate the basic habits which were perhaps laid out in the ancient school of wisdom in Mohenjo-daro, and Harappa almost two thousand years ago. Indeed, the human civilization has lost track instead of growing consciousness. The minds are stuck with endeavour, to succeed in the market place, and everything is being commoditized including women and love. Nature will showcase and empower in a negative way if you work against it, based on the **CAUSE and EFFECT** theory."

Martin,

"Do you know love is true? You are in a constant monologue inside. It is just on the surface. Perhaps her specific attitude has attracted you! Would you change your spouse often with her changing attitude. Perhaps it is a lot easier to change yourself!

The real image of the character of male or female is not looked at consciously in a state of awareness. If you're shrunk inside, how would you comprehend Nature in you and her. Then, How can you claim the better half will fit your bill. You mind is in a state of flux, and the next moment, someone looks beautiful! You have so many things conditioned by the media, so as your woman. Perhaps the woman in a man's mind is virtual, and no one can fit the bill. You anticipate your spouse to fit the bill.

How is this possible? In my view, the conditioning has poisoned every male. Perhaps women are heart centric by Nature, with emotional well-being. Mostly, Men are centric towards the head and hypocrites, whilst women are centered at the heart centre.

The entire India seems to have confused its heritage, and youth are changing, without knowing what to embrace, despite the cultural heritage of Yoga systems and meditation available a plenty. The irony is that some of them have been commercialized. You got to watch out the best one that suits you based on the personality.

Martin, It is easy if you will practice. Pick up any situation and practice AVR Technique. **Analyze-Visualize** and **Realize.**"

"Thanks Dr.!" Martin walks away, prepared to take more responsibilities of his life.

You've mastered the first four rules of 7 Golden Rules of Zen Wisdom:

> **Identify the 'SENSATIONS';**
>
> **Look 'BEYOND' the Sensations;**
>
> **Enjoyment in 'MODERATION';**
>
> **Identify the 'CONDITIONING' and AVR Method to resolve conflict.**

In the next workshop, you'll learn about the MIND and LINEAGE to GOD.

End of Session # 8

●●

4

The Mind Science

Day 8 – Session # 9:

Let's examine Self, Mind and its lineage to Eternity.

Rule # 5: Realize self, mind and lineage to Eternity

Martin was there on time for the next session. Dr. Richard continued...

"I would like to start off with a video of an inspiring tree."

"Ok. Dr. I am ready!!!"

The video was very inspiring as both watched without leaving a second.

Anecdote – The Wisdom Tree

"A little boy in 3 yrs. old was playing with the tree. And the tree started enjoying his companion. And she expected him to play everyday, and she started talking to him."

Boy: Mother, I just stay nearby. I love playing here.

Tree: You are welcome my son. Anytime come here and ask me if I can help you with something.

Boy: Mom, I need a cricket bat to play.

Tree: "You may break the branch and then use it to play as she gave a nice willow to play."

Boy: Oh Mom, thank you! he used the bat to play at school.

He began playing with the birds that have nests on the tree and the squirrels, all of them enjoyed their companionship. There was a snake!

Boy: Indeed, I am a little nervous Mom. Everything the little demon is looking at me. She is perhaps starring and snoring at me.

Tree: Oh come on, she is my pet, and she lives here, and it is her home. Don't worry, and she introduced her to the boy!

And the boy started playing with the snake and her family. It was joyful everyday, and it became his routine. Boy grew into a man. So as his desires.

Mom, "I am going away for higher education."

Ok. But please visit every year, she quelled with sadness."

"Of course Mom."

Once he came back to see her and then he returned back on overseas work.

Mom asked, 'how are you?"

Well. I need a job. Don't have time. Tell me.

He was in a hurry, Mom pampered him with her branches and leaves.

"What more can I give?" she asked. The Man never returned. After a while, he came back as a middle aged man with lots of ambitions!

"Mom, I just came back to see if you are there. Quickly need some bucks to start up my business."

"Ok. Good, my dear boy. What can I do?"

"Perhaps I can remove all the leaves to make some medicines as I have my friend who can help!"

Mom: Of course go ahead.

She became just bare branches with no leaves.

Wonder. Mom. "Yes."

"I made some money. Leaving overseas to setup my operations, he walked away without listening her whispering heart."

A middle aged man is now old man as he returned to the tree home.

"I love you! Where have you been?" Mom says.

"Mom, I was busy. Marriage, family etc."

"Good. You never sent me any message.

Man: I forgot, Sorry!

Mom: Ok. Well. What's up now?

Man: I am diseased, looking for some help from you.

Mom: Oh no, my dear son. What can I do to help you?

Man: I need the root to use it for the herbal medicine.

"Can I cut your branches?"

"Of course, son," the response came in spontaneously; but perhaps need you to be aware that I love you my son.

He brought in his friend Nick to chop the tree into pieces.

Nick: The trick worked. Well. Let us export roots to India for medicines, and the remaining to the East coast for some quick bucks.

Man: Ok. Nick. I am glad she agreed.

The heart was still there lying in the roots. She whispers. I have a secret to tell you. Oh my dear son, can you hear me my love? My dear son!

He was busy counting the dollar bills.

Her heart continues to whisper. Oh my son, Oh my son…

"I just stumbled upon billions of worthy Golden treasures hidden underneath the roots by Emperor Edward, which I wanted to tell you long back when you came here Just wanted to tell you when you were a little old and listening. But you never relent to my whispers. How may I handover these treasures buried under the roots."

The movie had an impact in Mr. Martin, he was touched by the spirit of the mother-tree!

Dr. Richard continued…

"The man wasn't listening to the heart. He threw the roots into the nearby river. The tree-mom had reached the destiny, after sailing across a thousand miles."

"Interesting." Martin nodded.

"Martin, Do we ever realize the hidden treasures? You do not need to be a PHD to realize the values of a human being with evolving consciousness."

"Don't you think it is possible to limit the Desires, Emotions etc."

"Yes, it is."

What do you expect more than that? Just think over and re-prioritize your "Thanks giving weekends" to celebrate it with the parents and the family get-together.

Martin, Think about the younger days, when you were in a school. The times of sharing with the neighbors, friends etc. in the high school, college. **How much are you missing now by running over mundane things in life, which is going to end at some point?**

Dr. continued without a break….

"Didn't you know about 'Alexander the Great?'"

"Oh yeah, read about World History."

When Alexander the great was about to die. He said '**Keep my both arms open before my funeral**' let the whole World understand that 'Alexander the Great' had nothing to carry.

You were born without anything; you were absolutely naked as pure consciousnes and now you carry one thousand and one thoughts, desires, emotions, sensations, genetics etc. Just drop it all and merge with the consciousness right now.

"I would like you to feel the moments and how much you have been blessed to be alive."

Often you regret the past moments, wasting the present moments too and ultimately you will regret the lost life! This is how your mind tricks you, hankering over the past or future moments!!!

"Martin, stop thinking. Just be where you are. Listen to the songs of the birds. Drinking tea is spiritual."

Martin interrupts…"I never thought drinking tea is spiritual."

"Yes, it is. In Zen, monks drink tea in totality in a state of no-mind. By simply being in totality."

"Interesting. I see what you are saying."

"You are born happy, and you were trained to be miserable." Enlightenment is your birth-right, and your consciousness does not carry any guilt. Mind is not a time machine, and you cannot be using without knowing its potential. If you are engaged externally by keeping the mind busy and thinking only in solving logical problems. It will frustrate you at some point! Perhaps you are using a flying machine for riding like a bullock cart!

What are you thinking about Mind? You will need to give out the due attention to analyze conditioning in the subconscious mind which is often surfacing to the conscious mind. Perhaps it will take the revenge to the core of the being if you aren't paying attention.

You have to drop the conditioning and nothing else. Perhaps this is the only thing that you'll need to renounce and not anything else to achieve eternal peace. As you seek truth out of your heart, you'll slowly feel peaceful and love filling your heart. It will be given to you at the right time, but the only fact is that you should seek out of the heart and look for the Divine intervention. Each of you carry this hidden treasure, which need to be realized. Unless you turn inward to the heart, the journey of consciousness will not happen. You'll remain stagnated!

Once you are focused more a little closer to the heart to find the deep awareness. Finally you will be able to realize the inner consciousness, which is the essence of it all; do not enter into the cyclic pattern, learn from the past conditioning and move on!

There is no point in hankering over the past as you're wasting the present moments; be happy by heart with love as the negative emotions will melt away. As you merge with the supreme consciousness, you will find the way to the uninterrupted bliss and the journey of micro-consciousness will reach its destination.

You are endowed with the capacity to perceive Nature itself as manifestations in the evolutionary process of Nature is human Mind; Perhaps an Ocean cannot perceive itself as an Ocean. Every moment is a mysterious, and it is revealing something to you, like the tree-mom. It is whispering into your ears right now. You should have the willingness to listen, be patient to hear the sounds of eternity.

The only way to listen to your heart. It is a science, as '**Mind is Wave**'. A deep psychological cleansing is required by self-counseling. Once you get over all past conditioning, the karmic-debts, you will be able to reach the subtle state of mind. In that state of static impressions, God will express in absolute silence. The identity of "I" will melt away, which is the ultimate state of **Enlightenment**.

Have you heard about the most successful person in your view those rich men are committing suicide? It is because of a sudden emptiness in their mind, as they do not know; There will be glimpses in mind, if you stop and listen. Just stop at times and relax deeply to find the hidden truth. Mind will start cherishing it to you.

You will be able to regain the lost creativity, and enjoy every moment. Instead, if you are stuck in constant chat outside; by and by mind will break down with the consequences of nervous break-down. May be it will result in schizophrenic split, landing you in an asylum.

Just be aware of the wonders, tap the inner potential and let the mind being used as a tool in the journey of the consciousness. You will be one with the Universe. This will be the beginning of a new life.

It is like a newly and happily married couple with the senses tied like a knot to the consciousness, and the micro-consciousness merged with the macro-consciousness. Life will blossom in to multitude of blissfulness!!!

Every success starts with a small step; this is a beginning of your successful life ahead, whatever way you have led your life. Just drop it along with the past conditioning. Let's move along hand in hand by helping each other in a commune. Perhaps the commune of the current and future generations to one commune.

"Martin, enough of a theory. Let me get on to work!"

"I need you to follow my instructions carefully."

"Ok. Dr."

Dr. asks Martin to lie down on a couch with dimmed lights and soothing music of Beethoven.

Dr. continues with his instructions:

"Relax your Body, Mind and Spirit. Breath in deeply-and Breathe Out-Be closer to the sensations of a trauma experiences

101

in the childhood-Be aware-Let the sensations of pain pass away and its melting. You are stronger now. Thank yourself for all the efforts that you have taken to come out of addictions successfully. Let it go!"

"Martin, Do contemplate for a while. Let the whole being enjoy the success that you have enjoyed in getting over an emotional state. And let this be alone your thinking point for the day, to build the character of strength and personality."

Martin, I am going to teach you about the functioning of mind in the next session, be ready!

Mind Functions

There are several instances of disorders in the psychiatry journal. Phobias, hallucinations are a typical situation of creating fear, anxieties and sleeping disorders or addictions with a repetitive pattern. These disorders are primarily due to lack of analysis, and the lost touch with the heart. As you keep cramming in so many of the information, you became a logical thinker. May be true that you would have scored well, but if you do not understand the feelings and emotions, you will tend to repress it deep in the unconscious mind.

Each of it would gain immense power, and surface in the conscious mind when it finds sometime this is based on my experience, and research, and each of it would gain enormous power. Even if you meditate, it will not sublimate as the power can be misused to divert the energy towards negativity. I'd call it as a particular situation in mind in a '**EXCITED**' state. This will create a trend in mind. This trend will create a cyclic pattern; thus creating an addictive behaviour.

Hence, you should analyze the roots of each of these emotions in deep silence and uproot it entirely by counseling in the state of meditation and peace. Each of these trends will be set in mind as patterns, thus influencing the behaviour and personality.

The senses work in tandem with the subconscious mind independently, superseding the conscious mind. As a result, you would feel pain due to excessive utilization of the senses. These additions to the taste, becomes a master, and the conscious mind is sidelined. In a similar analogy, sexual gratification or over indulging, or addictions are primarily due to the additions to the sensuality that you have perceived and addicted to it; It is like catching the tail of an elephant for happiness, without realizing the trunk.

The respective organs will take control over the mind, and thus resulting in a repetitive pattern of mind with energy wasted. These senses with the semi-conscious state can supersede mind; if you supply power to the conscious mind, it will gain enormous power and wisdom to regain the lost consciousness. This is the pattern of the mind functioning, and its conditioning.

A ZEN poem about MIND:

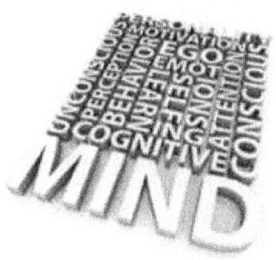

Mind is a Mind is a Mind,
Men may come, and Men may go,
I go on forever!!!

Perhaps none can stop as I will stop
On the day of judgment!!!

I'll collect whatever you did,
And react back hitting your consciousness;
You repent for nothing as a victim,
I play the spoil sport when you don't realize;

When intelligent men transcend,
By not finding the recordings of artifacts;
Perhaps realizing the heart, which is the Nature,
I am just a flux of the static truth at the heart!

I am the periphery,
Just a bubble as I am ready to burst!

Oh poor men,
Realize not that I am,
As I do not exist!
Only the state of flux as wave!!!

The moment you realize,
I burst open like a bubble burst,
To find the yielding love,
As the centre of your consciousness, will reveal!!!

I wish you finding the truth;
As I am the split called Mind,
Perhaps you conditioned me not,
Through millions of years in evolution!

Thou, not finding the Divine,
At the centre of the wagon wheel,
Seek me not, perhaps the Divine Nature;

Who is the observer, and the observed?
Find yeah the truth beneath the clouds,
Find the bright sunshine yet revealed!

The one who is realized through the focus,
At the centre of the wagon wheel,
Touch me not,
Heal me not,
Just be aware of the heart,
I'll exist no more!!!

Are these sensations real in a Mind?

Perhaps you may exclaim about Mind as sensations are not real. Even the real ones are in a state of flux, an excited state of energy either due to the urge from the physiology or created by you or even extending manifestations of thoughts. Each of these sensations, emotions are stored as dual strands in a split personality. The result is that you will hanker either way, and go between the extremes of either sides. The reason is that you have conditioning in the semi-conscious mind, which is not treated. And the condition in the conscious mind is a virtue.

There is always a constant conflict in mind to follow virtues in one side and the other side is exactly reverse. But whenever energy is endowed with goodness; there is a parallel line and a storage in the subconscious mind, which is proportionately growing due to lack of treating the karmic-debts.

You will not grow spiritually, unless you get rid of the karmic debts. These desires are need based. For example, food is a need when you are hungry. The need based food extended to the sensual enjoyment of "taste". You've become addicted to the senses eventually. This is the cause of all miseries as you were addicted to the senses, and the senses started controlling the mind. The simple analogy is eating food even if you aren't hungry at all!

The power of mind is constantly diluted. A particular event looks terribly satisfying, and eventually these situations of happiness will turn sour at some point. A deep realization is required, and senses should be alive but as an agent receiving commands from the mind. Then by and by slowly the mind power will increase, which can be harnessed towards spirituality.

When a Zen master asked a disciple:

Boju said, "get me some water."

"Ok. master, Hung Wei walked with a bucket."

105

He fetched some water from the well and walked back to the monastery which is half a mile; and the master laughed saying, you don't have water here.

It is all drained through the holes in the bucket and again he tried covering few holes. And it did not help.

"Just stop this nonsense, you are tired" Boju hit him gently to make him aware and said.

"Just plaster the holes. And fetch it now!"

"Simple as he quelled." And smiled at the master!"

The mind has been conditioned, with several pores open. Each of these pores has made you an addict through the senses. This is a trick played against humanity by the politicians, and the businessman. This is the cause of all miseries, anxieties, and disorders as you may call. And each of the wellness clinics to help you come out, whilst the food court's make you overeat by serving mouth-watering food!

First, society is responsible for overfeeding by constantly conditioning you through the senses, and sex has been made a taboo showing women in the poorest light from a soap opera to the sandwich maker and everything looks sexy in the view of masses; a lot of imported conditioning in the social hypnotism, leading you to miseries. Now, you understand the conditioning in the subconscious mind. The next step is to transform the conditioning by intellectual enquiry and reasoning.

When I heard of one of my colleague had passed away due to heart attack, my heart felt miserable. And for a moment, I realized there is nothing called '**PERMANENT**'. Though it sounds philosophical, you don't know what Nature has in store for you the real next moment. The Divine Nature has manifested in the mind. Nature will detach the soul from the body, as 'DEATH' to alleviate all your pains. The story of life is eternal, even if you die which is just a physiology; Nature will attach the soul to another body with a similar mind pattern

106

and karmic-debts in order to help you dissipate the karma's by the law of Nature. It is a simple science of wave theory, attuning right wave in the respective frequency.

The objective of life is to live through; enjoy it in moderation, and surrender to the Nature by realizing its inherent qualities and sublimate. There is nothing enjoying food or sex, but be awake and enjoy it to the core without leaving a trail of the moment in the past. If you understand the sensations, you will be surprised the same pattern is repeating over and over again with the same set of consequences in your body, mind and spirit. **"Then who is experiencing?"**

As we discussed sensations are achieved through the senses, whilst most of them are false sensations. Perhaps the purpose of GOD providing you ability to think, is to streamline your thoughts based on experiences. The observer and the observed are one and the same!

"Mind is a Wave", so as thoughts are and the sensations are shadow wave. Indeed these thoughts cannot sustain longer. It is like a ripple! May be you are fuelling it more and more by thinking about it and enjoying the fake-sensations. **"Have you observed?"** In silence, it would be so obvious that you are making it up with the 'negative' moods, and you hang and date with the sarcastic moods, which will end up in all sorts of frustrations. You aren't gaining any intelligence over the past cyclic pattern of thought!

The purpose of mind is to understand the value of this instinctive behaviour, and the conditioning of human conscious based on the four prime pattern of characterization such as 1) Quantity and Quality of the Sexual Vital Fluid, 2) Country and 3) Genetics. These factors would influence the way you think, behave and act upon. For example, West is predominantly analytical, it is research oriented, and East is predominantly from the heart centre in terms of feelings. Therefore, each context of excellent or hurtful is based on the baseline condition, which would vary.

The inevitable reasoning is required to develop a reliable baseline through the inner revelations of truth by your own practices. The cultural evolution is no longer accepted by science, and you will need science to prove every instance of religious practices; when science becomes your acceptance personally, and socially it will lead our lives of truth with reasoning including philosophy.

"Mind is just a wave."

"Dr. Please explain." Martin asks for more clarity.

"Ok. A simple analogy is that it can travel in time as you imagine the past events precisely, and it can record anything that you perceive through the senses. You are functioning like a bio-computer, with the capacity to view the centre as consciousness."

Dr. Richard draws few circles on the board.

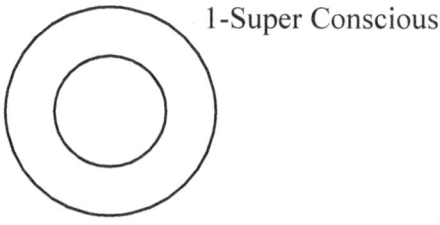

1-Super Conscious

The centre of mind is the intelligence, a pure state of consciousness as a gift of the Nature, and the periphery is the conditioned-mind, and the reactive Nature which is also Nature's gift, which is due to the evolutionary process from the single sense to the sixth sense. The centre is static, and the periphery is dynamic, like a wave and the ocean. The dynamic is mind, and the centre is super-consciousness or God.

As per Einstein's theory of relativity, World has concurred electrons **'WAVE NATURE'**. All particles are spinning with extremely high velocity, so is your life-force particle, the fundamental particles which forms your body. These particles with high velocity forms magnetic wave called **'MIND'**.

The centre is **'CONSCIOUSNESS'** and the **OUTER** is **WAVE 'MIND'**. It has the capacity to realize sensations based on the differences in the circuit.

The WAVE MIND will need to be streamlined from a state of flux to subtle wavelength. On the contrary, if you are in a state of over excitement continuously, you will feel disturbed as the magnetic variance in the circuit can impair the senses and neurons. This would result in losing ability to think, analyze, by depleting the mind power. A simple analogy is an electric circuit; if the consumption is as per the design, there will not be any short-circuit. In case, the water heater is consuming more than the designated units of power; then it will damage the coil inside, resulting in a short-circuit. This is exactly what happens in your bio-magnetic circuit. The over-usage of senses beyond the specific limit will breakdown eventually.

The mind power is enhanced in meditation as the magnetic circuit is closed, and you feed the energy back, thereby improving the mind power; The mind power can be harnessed for higher spiritual purposes by completing the circuit. As discussed in the above analogy, your senses are like 'equipments' that will utilize the magnetic units and transform into the respective sensations. If you exceed the conversion of magnetic units/second, then it will result in an over consumption beyond the specific limits.

"Martin, I've read the entire Hindu epic, Ramayana, an interesting one with my analogy of the demon king's conditioned MIND."

If you fuel all desires with the mind power, it will be lost in the drain as indicated in the Hindu Epics. In the Hindu epic of **Ramayana**; 'Ravana' is the Demon King of Srilanka who captures **Rama**'s wife, Sita, due to immoral passion! Ravana was taken a captive on the last day and Rama gives him a final ultimatum to release his wife, and surrender with an apology. The last ultimatum:

"Leave the battlefield today, and come Tomorrow."

– Ramayana

The last ultimatum of Rama is significant as he gives him a chance to reflect on Ravana's conditioning, and the consequences till date. But he refuses to realize his self, despite facing the consequences of losing the battle, kingdom and brothers etc. You do not find amidst reflecting the sensations and moods arising. And you tend to hold on to the 'tail', which are all sensations. Hence your mind seems to be complicated. The only way is to be centered, and focus at the centre of the mind itself, which is the Divine Nature.

Ravana was not all that bad except for his immoral passion and he is an ardent instrument player known as '**Yaazh**' in the East, synonymous to the modern day Violin. He had intensely practiced it in devotion, and a devotee of Lord Siva, whenever he composes music and songs even the Lord of the heavens descend, listening to his compilations. The fact is that, there is none called 'bad' or 'good'; You react to the past condition!

One of the six temperamental moods has not been treated in my opinion, which has surfaced from Ravana's semi-conscious mind. Being labeled a demon king, who are reactive by Nature! May be he was not capable of realizing the **CAUSE and EFFECT** theory; he was not in a subtle state of mind (frequency) to accept virtues since, he was possessed completely by the conditioned mind in the form of '**Kama**', which is the lower instincts. In another connotation, it reflects the lineage of '**Kama to Rama**', whilst, '**Kama**' indicates your lower instincts and '**Rama**', the highest evolution of consciousness.

These sensations are based on the need and thus, six temperamental moods are subjective to fulfilling the basic needs. When the need becomes greed, and desire the problem starts. For example, food, shelter are all basic needs if it extends beyond, then it becomes a desire.

110

The cumulative karmic debts aggravate the situation if thoughts are lying dormant in the unconscious mind are not achieved to fullest; it may empower you negatively at any moment. Like the star wars, you are overpowered by the Robots, which would eventually destroy the humanity. This is a similar situation; the energy of sex could kill you if you do not comprehend the energy. If you repress, the anaconda will express and eat you all. Anger can be controlled temporarily; if it explodes it will endanger self and the family. And the consequences are realized only after that you should go to the bottom of anger to comprehend truth.

In my view, these emotions are manifestations of the same energy in either North bound or South bound. '**How much you are able to harness it towards a successful life?**' To me success is not just the career; it is a multidimensional personality of heart and simplicity that you will abide knowing the facts of energy without having to hide your repressions. When you become extremely aware in the moment, and transcend it instead of repressing with a smiley face in front of the community in a church! An empty discipline or a goal is dangerous as you will achieve occasionally. The underlying energy will try to escalate in another dimension.

The real power of harnessing the inner transformation is lying on the energy moving upward in the Northward bound. How manyof it have you harnessed it intellectually for the spiritual growth? God has given you the power to contemplate past events, and understand the karmic debts, and move on, as you cannot simply drop the whole past overnight behind the inherited over thousands of years. It takes time to understand, analyze and move on in spiritual practices. Nature has evolved in over millions of years, finally manifesting as the human consciousness!

God wanted you to realize the entire background, study the artifacts of sensations; rationalize as pain or peace or happiness and find out the reasons through your inquisitiveness mind. The capacity of mind is the ability to take any shape, and it becomes the object that you think, with its consequences. The moment you think about eternal consciousness itself inpurest form, you are advancing towards something eternal, in everlasting peace and blessedness of truth.

The mind has the capacity to expand in North bound or South bound, unlike your non-behaving market trading, it is fluctuating a little less if you realize it by way of conditioning.

North

South

The irony is that you can fuel it either way. And meditation can help you to accumulate the energy. And only through the introspective analysis and centering process, you will be able to counsel yourself on the reality behind every sensation to divert the negative pattern or behaviour into positive Northbound home.

The Supreme consciousness is yielding in love, and constantly teaching in each of the endeavour. The social, psychological values are formed based on the imprints. The link will attract similar pattern to dissipate the karmic debts. Each of you is blessed with a spouse in the first place, whom you never realize; the other one is none other than the reflections of the inner core and the surface which is trying to uncover itself.The wholeplay is intended to teach you something, to teach you about the Divine blessings, to help you reclaim the lost consciousness, and help you to reach home as the light is inside you.

Buddha often said '**Be a light unto you.**'

'**Appo deepa bava**'

You have to listen to the songs of the heart, and enjoy your time in silence and thank for the benediction and blissfulness; In one of the Hindu Epics of **Mahabharata**, the entire story is due to the greed and desire of Duriyodhana in the Kurukshetra war of deadly battles ever in the history. It is due to Dhuri's greed and desire for wealth, in a conditioned-mind set.

'Martin, I felt inspired by Hindu epic, Mahabharata, which had helped me in the analogy of conditioning. My theory papers have reached Mr. President's office for the upcoming World Religious confluence, where I am going to talk about the conditioned mind with inferences from Hindu epics, Ramayana and Mahabharata!'

"Dharm had lost his kingdom in a card game. As agreed, he completed fourteen years in the forest, and he returns back to claim his kingdom as agreed. However, Dhuri, who was conditioned negatively for selfish desire by his maternal uncle Sakuni, denied his kingdom."

"My dear brother, Gone are the days of anger. I just want to live peacefully through the rest of my life with my brothers and family. Please handover my kingdom back to me," Dharm claims.

Dhuri: "No."

"Would you allow me a small portion of the North East of the barren lands for us to lead?"

Dhuri: "No way," he looked at his uncle 'Sakuni'.

Dharma: "Ok. Well, give me at least a palace to stay for the family. A home for us as we do not have anywhere to go."

"Well said my boy," Sakuni clapped his hands.

Dhuri: "No, I cannot give you even a single cent of land. Go away."

The above scenario indicated Dhuri's conditioning, perhaps he would have been aware! He was conditioned by his uncle, Sakuni.

Dhuri was not all that rubbish, once he saw the ability of swordsmanship in Karna, who was a formidable warrior.

Immediately he greeted him with open arms, and awarded the land to him though for his personal gains of adding strength to his army. He willingly admitted through his friendship, and camaraderie looking at the plight of Karna who is the best in archery, and had the ability to beat anyone in the battle including Arjun.

I would say it is all because of conditioning, and the **IDEALISM** is based on the conditioning; on what and how you were taught in the past. Hence, these beliefs that you have had till date is either communicated by the Religion, parents or inherited from the society, however none of it is realization based, as you have not felt anything as the inner revelations.

The only way to get over the past conditioning is to reflect deep enough, and get over the past through inner revelations in the meditative state of mind. There is no other way to change the old pattern of habits, and there is no need for a primal therapy. All you need to do is to keep engrossed in the moment to moment awareness.

Mind has the ability to introspect, which is one of the unique quality of Mind; as you can go back in Time think about a situation, and heal them. Perhaps this would help you superimpose the conditioning, with virtues that you actually feel by heart. The repressed emotions, feelings would surface to the consciousness. Though you might have achieved success economically, spiritually these thoughts could cripple you at a split second. You would be terribly surprised to observe all that you've received, recorded and conditioned till-date, is based on your perceptions of short-sighted one dimensional (1D) view.

It needs patience to realize and reveal one dimensional (1D) perspective into two dimensional (2D), and consequently a three dimensional (3D) view to transcend beyond all these conditioning. Otherwise life would prove to be a waste of time, and eventually you would run out of steam one day when you retire. These thoughts will surface at some point when you are alone. A real successful person is the one who is capable of remaining absolutely silent, cherishing in moments of silence. enjoying alive in every moment to moment awareness. Anything you do is not going to help, and money cannot buy peace of mind or eternal bliss. It is required to fulfil basic needs!

If you are in an emotional state of mind, in 'BETA' state of Mind, which indicate the frequency of the mental wavelength, then you are influencing the thoughts of lower value. This is due to the fact that you inadvertently attract forces of negative energy. The power of cosmic consciousness supports both positive and negative; and augments with the super-conscious mind, depending on what you attune. Though the inner conscience guides to centre, the outer will attract based on the conditioning.

You'll tend to work outwardly for pleasures, with no understanding of the origin of these sensations which are packets of energy in mind. If the expenditure is more, the disorder is more in mind. Hence, there is displeasure in everything you do. The perceptions are based on your conditioning. You may hanker for food, or sex or perhaps even more addicted through the sensual pleasures.

Now ask a question if all of that is external stimuli or internal, you are ready to bounce at any moment. If you are angry, no matter who is in front of you? Either you repress or express. The bottom line is that anger is residing within subconscious mind, and sex is there lying dormant, waiting for an opportunity.

These are just the manifestations of energy and Nature is unconditional love, as it helps you with ways to heal the conditioning. It is bound by "TIME-DISTANCE-VOLUME-FORCE" which are the four dimensions of wave, the 'Mind Wave'. The law of Nature governs every aspect in life from a simple atom to the Galaxies with precision.

The mind can travel by the process of thinking, and it can take any shape. It can defy 'TIME; as you can go back and forth in thoughts, isn't it? The mind in expansion becomes a Super Conscious mind, with the only difference of the body as a boundary.The conditioning has been imported to you, through utilizing the senses subconsciously and it takes a lot of effort to dissipate whatever you have observed.

Even animals are not excited through conditioning. They are instinctive as discussed, and there is no animal worried about the face creams. Did you ever notice birds copying the dream girl? It is funny the way human consciousness has scattered in hallucinations in the form of nudity in art!

The urge is to unite, which is perhaps natural, but you have been conditioned to hold on to the sensations. There seems to be poisoning at the roots of sexual energy. This resulting in corrupt senses and the crooked thinking; The pursuit of human consciousness is to achieve happiness, which is the goal, but perhaps somewhere it is stagnated without evolving any further.

You will need to analyze each of your temperamental moods at the grass root level, and you will be surprised to find a 2-D view of each of it, and your sexual energy is perhaps due to a childhood repressions, or anger is something due to a desire to excel and the social conditioning by looking at others. Each of the moods fluctuations; are predominantly due to factors such as:

1. **Need based,**
2. **Habitual,**
3. **Circumstances,**
4. **Social, and**
5. **Genetics**

Each of your thought is classified into one of the above. The conditioning can be analyzed. For example, a deep desire to become an Engineer or a Doctor is perhaps Genetics like your father. Or addictions to drinking are due to social by friends or someone else at work.

There may not have a real need for food, rest or sex, despite being fulfilled by the bodily urge. Perhaps you may not be hungry for food, but you still go to a restaurant due to habits.

These habits are plentiful and lousy! Eventually, you become habituated and addicted. An addiction can take you far away from the centre, and perhaps with no possibilities of returning back home. Be aware.

'Enough of theory. Martin, I'll let you practices something very simple.'

Dr. Richard hands him over a pen and paper handy!

'Ok. I'll give you 3 minutes to identify the thoughts that are passing by now.'

Martin starts writing something on paper. "Ok. Now, go-ahead and identify each of these thoughts and contemplate."

Scale Of Mind

"Martin, Now, let's watch something, a fable for you."

"Didn't you realize the scale of Mind seems to be changing every second from a car, house, so on and so forth."

"Is it wrong?" Mr. Martin enquiries.

"Hmmmm. It is not wrong, but greed could lead to limitless desires of eternity, which could possibly drain your energy into temperamental moods. You should focus on what is possible, without deviation from the final Goal. May be you should not compare constantly with others, in terms of material wealth as you are endowed with eternal being as mind and unique design. God wants you to scale up."

"The ultimate expansion is the final scale to realize in mind, and there is no need to feel disappointed by comparing with someone who has achieved some mundane wealth based on the efforts and karmic-debts."

"Everyone should realize this, and futility of comparing with others is not going to help. Didn't you realize your uniqueness? You have the ability to change. There is no reason to be antagonistic against anyone or with you for not being able to achieve a similar feat as that of others."

"It is your Nature to compare; unless you expand it to the consciousness to find yourself eternal as it is your intrinsic Nature."

Here is another anecdote for you, Martin:

"A disciple was meditating deep in the forests for years, for a boon in life."

God intercepted finally after finding his convictions. **'My Son, I am proud of your meditation and convictions towards me.'**

"What do you want?"

The long beard Sadhu opened his eyes slowly.

Worshipping Lord. Asking him to give him the powers to convert everything to Gold!

Everything looked beautiful to the Sadhu. He was able to convert iron pieces to Gold. He had mastered the alchemy of gold, and he became the richest man in the town!

He had everything, but he could not enjoy food or relationship. He went back.

"God, I cannot enjoy food."

"You take these powers. I want to live with powers of becoming the most powerful man in town."

"So you have it," God exclaimed!

He became the minister and after a while he was fed up with the ministry as nothing was fulfilling and there was a void in his heart, as everything seemed political with people respecting upfront and plotting him to murder him by envying him and he lost his sleep.

He goes back to the forest. "Meditating."

"God, please help me. You take the powers back. I do not need anything."

"Well. So be it". God said in the reverberating voice behind Sadhu and a stream of light passing by!

He went back to farming. And he enjoyed simple life, and he was married, happily cherishing moments. It was not anusual palatial bungalow. He liked his new hut, which was very peaceful with the moon intercepting every month.

Now, he was sitting quietly, doing nothing!

His kids and wife had gone out for a neighbors wedding.

God intercepted him. And asked him.

"Oh Sadhu. Well. Do you have anything to ask?"

"God, Thank you! I have nothing to ask as I am not the same man who was in the forest with desires to achieve anything."

"I just want to say "THANK YOU" for what you have given my Lord. And why didn't you say this at the beginning?"

"My son, You're unique in the World. I created you to feel by your inner revelations." And you have Mind which the tool is provided to you.

God speaks, "Sadhu, I have come to ask you for something."

"What? For a change" Sadhu exclaims in remorse!

"How can I help you and what do I feel that you do not have?" Sadhu asks.

Your mind has evolved; with the capacity to expand, and realize self and the supreme consciousness. You are the ultimate expression of Truth. I cannot experience from the outside. Perhaps you have the capacity to comprehend, as revelations and hold me deep inside.

"Now, I want to feel the eternity, through you. May I borrow your mind?"

"Oh my GOD!" Sadhu actually exclaimed. And says:

'By all means'

This is a beautiful story which indicates revelations of truth. The **"MIND"** is the ultimate, and it can expand beyond what you may remember as it is eternity itself. You have been endowed with this truth, reality and beyond which you can expand, unite with cosmos and realize the evolutionary process. This completes the cycle, and even God in my view, does not have the ability to think. As it is a pure consciousness.

Eternity, Time and Consciousness as factors and mind are "you" which can realize it all. Just ponder over it!

In simple terms, understand: **'The Other End of MIND is GOD'** You have conditioning from the Genetics of human and animal which has all cumulative experiences till-date, known as the karmic-debts. Everything that you do in time will help you to discover **Truth**.

You will understand every situation is trying to tell the truth and the consciousness within you! You will end up leading a miserable life if you fail to liaise with the Divine energy. Your senses will play the spoil sport. A deep realization to use the senses is required, as a master. Perhaps you should enjoy using the senses, but not hankering over it.

"Martin, Just reflect on this." Dr. continues:

Your life has been a trade and commerce so far. Mind is constantly involved in the process of thinking, action and reaction, nothing else. The consciousness is lost in oblivion. Your Mind power has been wasted beyond a limit, without awareness in a state of deep slumber. The only Facet is not to hold on to the emotions; just be an observer, perhaps you are watching a movie, be courageous to be an observer with no judgment.

"Think about your past 10 years:"

Your relationships/Marriages, parenting and wealth; A success or a failure depending on the context; The painful sensations or children, adolescent kids causing trouble, and a job loss or any experiences of the recent Trauma in your life; including loss of the loved ones, thus havoc in the life.

"Think about your past 20 years:"

You were in a college, work, first job, marriage etc. And the sequence of responsibilities. Perhaps love, and relationships that you have gone through so far.

"Think about your past 30 years:"

Perhaps you were in a school. Treated like a King by your parents and the birthday celebrations etc.

Do you realize now? It is all projections now. Nothing seems to be real. At times, you were a saint, and mostly feeling guilty so on and so forth. If you had meditated a little bit, perhaps it makes sense, and these memories would yield some truth, perhaps a taste of the divine, eternal.

Someone asked Buddha about his age. He said:

"I am 20 years old" when he was biologically 55.

He has termed his age from the day of Enlightenment. The real moments are the ones, when you were aligned with the superconsciousness; in yielding truths, and the actions that you have done in sync. On the contrary, anything you have done till now out of sync with Nature is just a sheer waste of time.

The clear thinking is required to reflect on the past condition. There is so much work required to maintain good health rest is required, and proper food is required for metabolism. The point is that anything done in moderation within the limits is spiritual, and in tune with the "**UNIVERSAL LAWS of CAUSE and EFFECT**". Anything you have done till date by exceeding the limits, resulting in painful sensations. This would result in unnecessary pain, suffering and miseries in life.

The purpose of life is to understand the inner self and transcend the sensory perceptions. And move towards the spirituality which is lying dormant within each of you. It is based on my experience, anything in life would result is futile experience after a while; and there is nothing to achieve in life except leading the way towards realization. Perhaps this is the only endeavour in life. And nothing will give you happiness, ecstasy and bliss in life.

Each of these instances will teach you something. If you reflect on the progress, and the failures which have a lesson embedded in it. And reflecting on these would help you get out of the cycle; the vicious cycle as you have been trapped. A deep psychoanalysis is required to get you out of the condition.

Reflecting on each of this conditioning is a primal therapy to seek truth beyond the conditioning as the outer is a little hard!!! when you break open the inner core, or the yolk is the inherent spirit.

This is one of the wonders in the tool offered by the mother '**NATURE**'. She does not have the ability to think retroactively, though she has manifested in the human MIND's and thinks through us. As an eternity, in that context she cannot think unless she becomes human!!!

In a way, you have been gifted with "**MIND**". Unfortunately, you have not realized it as a gift since no one has taught you about it. **Let's watch** an action movie, they break for a cup of coffee and back on-time to watch an action packed thriller!

Anecdote: 'One Night at the Amazon Forest:'

American glider aircraft crash landed amidst amazon forests deep. Somewhere in coastal Africa:

It was late in the evening:

"Screeeeeeeeeech…**May Day. May Day**," the pilot yelled and crashed landed.

"Oh my God, just got the bird down, damn it! We are alive. Halle luau!!! We are alive for Christ sake as the American Scientist lamented with a mild blow on his head."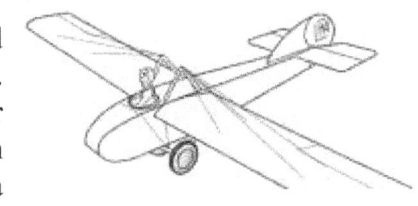

Both got down exploring the dense forest; with the chorus of wild animals from a distance. It was blazing sunlight in the morning woke up both American's with an unusual treatment.

"Vow vow, why are there so many seminaked men around here?" the second one exclaimed.

"Indeed. They are the aboriginals of this forest," replied the other.

"Ooooooohvuhhhhh" as a group of men bamboozled at these two Americans; pointing a spear at both of them; "you guys aren't going to hurt me? Do you?" asked the scientist.

"Oh no. These are smart fellows as the other one pacified with a fear in his blue eyes."

The head of the unit came forward, who was extraordinarily built with the muscles and rugged look with several beads tied around his head, forearms, carrying a large spear. He wore an ornament around his neck with few teeth of tiger with the shorts made of tiger skin.

"Man, he is terrific." one exclaimed;

"Just calm down," the other one said;

'Mumbo tumbo Hana Hana!!!'

"What the hell is that?"

Everyone started looking at the glider. And one of them was at the cockpit. "Shhhhhhhhhhhhhhh," Don't do that," the pilot screamed! Do not start the engine as the other one yelled.

One of them ran away to bring in few forest bulls, they Tied a few of these bulls with the cart in front ahead of the glider with a rope, and they started using the glider as a perfect bullock cart!!!

"This is how you are using MIND!!!" Dr. Richard concludes in the video.

"I cast this video a few years ago!!!!"

"Wonderful. Dr. You've done well! I like it. It's a Hollywood movie."

"True." May be not a fiction, it is intended to make you understand the values that you've been carrying.

While you can start a little bit by exploring, learn and fly to the shores of consciousness. You've limited to the senses, and cry for help later-on. What do you expect God to do, as he has already provided you the tool to find the route? You'll need to find the roadmap with the support of the inner conscience.

End of Session # 9

••

5
Mind Power

Day 9 – Session # 10:

The Mind Power Is Constantly Diluted

Perhaps, you aren't doing any action in the state of

awareness. Every action is a function of spending the mind power through the senses. There is a difference in you drinking tea Vs. Buddha drinking tea! And the reason is due to the state of mind in awareness. Therefore, you have a choice to be aware or not! Every action is performed by spending the mind-power. It will be diluted; hence there is a social need to perform an act in the state of awareness.

A simple evidence is watching a movie is perceived as sensation of pleasure by spending the energy through eyes or food that you taste by spending the mind power realized as sensations of taste! It is like a bank deposit if the 'CREDIT' balance (CR) increases you feel happy. When the energy levels rise above the critical level, you feel so filled in and energetic or the energy depleted below the minimum critical level is perceived as a state of depression!

On the contrary if the energy levels decrease due to the past conditioning and always in conflict with Nature, with actions in dual split resulting in expenses. If the expenses of the mind power go beyond a minimum critical level, it will cause all maladies in mind. If you trace your spending through sensations, you will be able to identify the root causes of the illness. It will result in thousand and one mental disorders. For example, Analyze sensations of excitement, anger and mood swings. You will be able to trace the 'REAL' Vs. 'FALSE' sensations, and discard the 'FALSE' sensations.

You keep moving between the varying length of mind; hence you are not sure whom you are. First, you act like a saint in the church, or a synagogue or a temple or mosque and then a sinner in the evening!

The same atom is responsible for a Gandhi, or a Mussolini. You can become a Mahatma, not just be following the principles of three monkeys, as knowledge will only repress the emotions. Deep down you will be hankering for happiness, and every time you say No, there is another strand of imprint deep down in the subconscious mind, which would eventually lead you to miseries. Though you may perceive success; the negative conditioning would come up with large sequence of negative consequences. The only way is to surrender to the vast eternity, which would heal you. You don't need to hold up all emotions in Ego, whereas a simple technique is to give up and surrender to the Divine Nature in love.

A simple analogy, '**When you dissolve a table spoon of salt in the sea, it just disappears in no time.**' This is a true based on my experiences! Your problems are minuscules, when compared to the cosmos. Perhaps you make it loud, and magnify the problems with the lenses. It is an ocean filled in blissfullness, you'll need to drop your identity "I" to merge with the cosmic truth.

Whatever you do, whoever you are, just dissolve into eternity, and that dissolution process of mind into the vast Eternity or darkness will '**HEAL**' you. There is no other possibility; A table spoon of salt will dissolve in the ocean, leaving no traces of negativity. The science has started listening to the philosophy for the first time in the evolution of human consciousness.

And the subsequent evolution will happen only through the consciousness; by linking science and philosophy, and there is no other possibility or no other magic pill can heal you or take you to the eternity.

You weren't thinking as a child holding the hands of your Papa! Isn't it? You entrust him so much, and you were tourning the entire city without a roadmap, by just following his footsteps. If it is possible for a child, then why can't you hold the hands of the eternal consciousness?

The past conditioning and karmic-debts will start shattering, and disappearing. Every particle is a wave nature. If it is true, '**Mind is a Wave**'; then the emotions are shadow wave emerging from the primary wave, like a ripple. It is imprinted in a startled state in the brain cells. When you think, which is replaying these thoughts in mind; it will excite the brain cells by creating a startled set of sensations or emotions causing mood fluctuations in each of you. This is the secret of Universal Magnetism and the inner Bio Magnetism. It functions in sync with laws of Nature. You can store an event precisely and "play" back along with sensations when needed. For example, when you think about an experience of trauma of the childhood, it appears true with the sensations of pain at any age in the lifetime! This indicates the wave nature of the mind which can store and play it back!

The **LAWS OF NATURE** works with the principles of (1) PATTERN, (2) PRECISION and (3) REGULARITY. Everything in the universe functions with orderliness from the smallest of the atom to the huge planets, galaxy. The primordial state is static manifesting into dynamic and further into elements, compounds and Galaxies etc. Finally in animate to the animate to the evolution of physical and mental-senses from single sense to five senses.

Finally, Nature has manifested as the human consciousness as '**MIND**'. The mind has the capacity to record everything precisely and replay as you may wish. There is some strong reason why Nature has endowed you with MIND being able to perceive pain, pleasure through the senses and peace. The sensations of pleasure or pain are due to dissolving the mind power in sensations.The consciousness is recording every event, and experiences as sensory enjoyment!

When you become addicted to the sensory perceptions, your mind is split as deep in the conscious it claims to be happy. For example, if you're drunk and have merry, everything seems beautiful which is an illusion, created by you, deep in the subconscious Mind. When you try that the next day, nothing appears, and it looks extremely stupid and irrational.

All your untreated fears, anxieties, nightmare, sensual pleasures are all stored in the subconscious mind which all would surface when you have enough energy restored. The one who is meditating for the first time would face a lot of waves of negativity emerging, and it is terribly disturbing initially until it settles down. But stay focused as GOD is on your side whenever you're trying abide by the LAWS OF NATURE. For every single step that you venture into realizing NATURE, It will help you in six steps towards the realization.

If this is your case, just let go as time passes it would heal and cannot stand along the way. Be aware and an observer. A night watchman who is aware and alert in every moment.

Buddha asked someone:

'Did you allow any unwanted guests?' They will drive the hosts one day, just identify these unwanted guests (thoughts) in the house of MIND, and do not greet them by heart. This is enough for guests who would not get enough attention to leave immediately.

This is exactly what I have realized in my life too. If you ignore unwanted thoughts; and counsel yourself with a little intelligence it would heal eventually with no significant repercussions. Otherwise, it will be there deep down as unwanted guests untreated or thought about, would suddenly emerging in your conscious layer driving you almost crazy.

'A little pinch of salt is enough to spoil a glass of milk.' In a similar way, a pinch of negativity is enough to cloud your consciousness mind, and the conditioning is exactly doing that. Your mind power is wasted by the strands of negative thoughts. You have to be aware of thoughts passing by, do not even diagnose initially as you got to witness.

When you restore energy and further by closing the pores of unwanted guests, the energy levels will increase with Oceans of bliss from everywhere. Your life will change forever with different perspectives.

Martin, I'll introduce you to the Management Guru, Dr. Maddy, A Leader of the spiritual empowerment, India with profound wisdom in management.

"Hello Dr. Maddy!"

"Hello Mr. Martin!" They chat for sometime over a cup of coffee.

Ok. We have few other participants waiting to hear from Dr. Maddy. Welcome Dr. Maddy from India for his services to humanity. He is here with us today to share profound wisdom and management philosophy to empower you.

Dr. Maddy speaks:

Thanks to you all and my pleasure being here with each of you. You may interrupt at any time during the session, as I would like to keep it an interactive session.

Dr. Maddy starts his speech on the stage:

"It is all based on the baseline conditioning, and interpretations. Did you notice animals don't get angry, and they are instinctive?"

He opens up the slide deck with topic "Managing Self and Empowerment."

Mind is a state of flux. Perhaps you are professionally managing at work, however, you fail to reckon the inner potential. The need of managing self is missing in the fast-paced World today, resulting in a split mind filled with confusion.

The "MAGIC QUADRANT" is a reflection of inner self. Each of it indicates the evolution of consciousness.

The following magic quadrant indicates the evolution of consciousness in to various stages:

Magic Quadrant

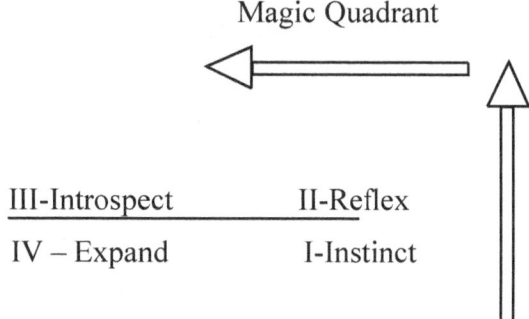

III-Introspect	II-Reflex
IV – Expand	I-Instinct

I – Instinct
II – Reflex
III – Introspect
IV – Expand

The primary instincts are common for humans; such as in animals and an urge to complete the instincts is quiet natural such as food, sex, rest and work. These are the basic instincts. The instincts will start based on a need such as sensation of 'hunger'. It is spiritual to dissipate the hunger, meaning sublimating the desire expands through the senses instead of sublimating urges by righteous means. The social responsiveness is to abide by the social setup, by evaluating the values and sentiments of the society.

The second quadrant indicates reflexes such as reactive behaviour, like the behaviour based on the reflexes. When the reflexive behaviour is not analyzed, it grows into a particular type of disorder. If not treated these reflexes can grow to a disorder including sexual disorders due to over excitement, involving the compulsive behaviour due to reflexive sexual passion.

The third quadrant indicates the introspective analysis of six temperamental moods. The power of the mind, consciousness and motivation in this quadrant to practice and achieve success as you will move to the either side of the emotional strings both Northbound and Southbound, and frequently escalating conditioning from the unconscious can possibly bother you.

You will need to surrender totally to the ultimate which would dissipate negative imprints;The one who is totally aware can adjudge good or bad based on the outcome based results. This is based on the evaluating against '**IDEALISM**' or principles of law of Nature to comprehend through the inner revelations. This will form your own principles, replacing these conditions; which can be evaluated in any state of mind.

The one who is clear with fewer thoughts and the senses in control is the one who has achieved success spiritually. Otherwise, you would keep on accumulating spiritual energy on one side and dissipate on the other side. The first step in this quadrant is to analyze the situation, visualize outcome based results and energize you towards positive results. The behaviour is changed entirely over a period of time, and your motive will remain in union with the Divine Nature.

The fourth and the final quadrant indicate the expanded state of mind without imprints. This indicates the state of eternal bliss, as they are sublimated with any further genetic imprints exist. An empty mind is a God's workshop who plays tunes through you.

Dr. Richard continues...

"Thank you Dr. Maddy." Any questions please.

Audience: "Sir, Please explain conditioning!"

Dr. Maddy responds: "It is all just the conditioning which is taking you out of the Divine Nature. May be you have forgotten the language of the heart, and ways to communicate within yourself."

Who is responsible, Dr.? Nature or Self?

Nature cannot be at her fault as evolution is her inherent quality, and the responsibility is lying dormant in you. Just observe a plant that flowers with effortless efforts, and the birds that sing in tune with the morning sunshine and the ease of everything which are most complex things from events of Earth and stars etc.

There should be the contentious process of evolution with a goal to realize your past conditioning, and the baggage that you have been carrying so far. If you let go without analyzing your behaviour, it will lead you to several consequences of lost life eventually in the path of miseries, anxiety, fear and deep split within yourself.

Well. The reason why human consciousness is endowed with mind is to help you visualize, analyze and comprehend to the truths. If it expands north bound it becomes **Rama** doing virtuously and it becomes **Kama** the god of sex in the south bound. It gets dissolved into condition. Mind and senses absorb or perhaps dissipate your energy of mind resulting in long term consequences of diseases.

The human minds have filled or replaced actions; towards survival either physically or mentally, and not to expand beyond! If the primary instincts are fulfilled, animals are in unison with Nature. Perhaps Nature is expecting humans to evolve beyond the instinctive mindset and realize all conditioning.

Perhaps this is the only challenge that God has imposed on you, and he helps you from every nook and corner from the chapel to the cathedral, it is ringing a bell in your mind in the form of love, truth, honesty as her intrinsic qualities. She keeps yelling from the roof top as a rooster to the moon, and the orgasmic unity is everywhere.

Whenever a bud blossoming into a beautiful flower, Sun and the moon and the stars all cherishing it happiness, except the human mind, which has forgotten the language of being in unison, neither through the instinctive mind nor by expansion. Once a while in every hundred years a saviour will blossom into his fullest defying all gravity of conditioning; and the Christ will once again be on the cross.

It is a cycle, and Nature will try again and again by helping consciousness to bloom whosoever is open and honest through the heart filled in love. You are filled in with emotions, and how else do you expect your pot to be filled; which is already filled in with emotions. The human consciousness is stalled due to negative emotions as you keep creating one thousand and one new events in mind with varying sensations. Everything is so natural, except human consciousness. But the basics of each of these moods remain in six temperamental moods.

Dr. Maddy continued to explain Mind Vs. Senses

Mind Vs. Senses

The mind is immensely powerful in the expanded state of consciousness. It is absolutely required to think rightly to avoid pains, as your desires can also grow eternally as your being has the only instinct of merging with the conscious. The mind will try to find bliss in the emotional state unconditionally; as the conditioning can side track due to the duality in mind. If the condition is not treated from the subconscious mind, it will play the spoil sport till the energy will be thoroughly drained away.

A simple analogy: When you make a path or channel through which water flows to the garden, it becomes typical whenever it rains, and water flows. In a similar context, mind will also form grooves to let the energy flow through the senses. Like music flowing through the instrument is nothing but air, your mind power (magnetic energy) will flow through the senses, and each sense has its consciousness thus feeling sensations in the respective organs equipped. Now, you will become addicted to the senses, rather than realizing it through the conscious mind. It is essential to ponder over your "**Mind Vs. Senses**". If you are a master, your consciousness will be the centre and the master equipping mind and the senses.

Conscious-mind-senses

Mind can be a slave to the Senses or a master, depending on how you intend to utilize. It is as simple as that, when you overengage a motor beyond its capacity, it fails. You have to know the limits of sensual pleasures, and enjoyment, and never allow senses to take over. It reminds me of a movie called spider man, where the robotic arms of the villain take control of his neurons. Simple analogies that will help you understand.

The evening session was even more crowded, someone in the crowd asked a question:

"Hello Dr. Maddy! I am Thompson."

"Hello, Thompson!"

"What is your question?"

"Dr., could you explain "**Satvic**" food as you call in India?"

"Sure." Dr. Maddy continued.

Food For Thought

Did you notice? "**Food influences sensations**". If you observe artifacts of eminent saints, scientists and leaders, there is one common trait that I have observed. A balanced diet to keep the body healthy, if you over eat, your body feels heavy; therefore, you will not be able to execute the analysis in terms of scientific or self-inquiry, both will need some deep mind being in a lower frequency to research.

Hence, in olden days say 2000 years ago, India had satvic type of food as they predicted food is your being, and food is what you are now. Essentially food becomes the following finally:

1. Juice
2. Blood
3. Fat
4. Bone Marrow
5. Flesh
6. Sexual Vital Fluid

If you consume red-meat, it affects your physiology. In psychological terms; when animals are slaughtered, they release hormones which are poisonous to the human body, and they carry imprints. Their behaviour is instinctive. Hence, you would also accumulate its behaviour. This is evident as a recent survey across countries. The recent survey indicates countries, where they eat red-meat have been identified with the maximum number of violence registered.

The assimilation of red-meat takes longer as your body is a sophisticated machine, which has been provided by Nature with the ability to cultivate food. In India, predominantly a sect of people succeeding in most of the endeavour such as arts, literature, music etc. If you analyze their food habits, it is a simple food, and milk, hence by Nature they have inherited a lower frequency by way of consuming only vegetarian food.

Also, remember overeating is harmful, as excess food is stagnated; this will produce more hydrochloric acid stimulation to digest.

As your system will be forced to digest, in that process a quanta of food will remain indigested. Causing your stomach upset. And all sorts of problems, with persistent behaviour it would lead to diabetes as it impacts the secretion of vital hormones. You have to be aware of produce from the Inorganic farming which is the usage of chemical fertilizers to grow produce. This is harmful in the longer run, and genetically modified seed which is one of the causes of cancer.

While west has improved in the medical science, a basic understanding of the sexual vital fluid is not evident as they deny the power of sexual vital fluid. They treat it as a fluid with some protein, fat etc. It carries your history in Genetic imprints till-date.

Dr. Maddy, what is sexual vital fluid and how is it linked to spirituality as highlighted in the Indian scriptures?

Dr. Maddy continued….The sexual vital fluid is the source of your life-force generated, which in turn produces biomagnetism which is required for conversion through the senses. A minimal stock of the sexual vital fluid is required to balance between body, mind and spirit. If it used for enjoyment by excessive behaviour, it will lead to diseases. The sexual vital fluid can be transmuted to spiritual energy through a specific breathing practices. This would enhance mind power.

Dr. Maddy, could you explain managing stress?

Managing Stress

You are aware of the harmful results of stress. If you do not manage it now, at an early age. Hence, it is imperative you focus on the daily schedule, prioritize what is essential in life with a balanced life-style thereby avoiding sedentary life-style and its results.

If you are overly stressed; you will have a nervous breakdown, a simple and profound practices of breathing such as 'NahdiShuti' can avert all of the harmful effects.

Let's do this:

A simple breathing technique to get rid of stress:

1. Breathe in deeply through the left-nostrils by closing the right nostril with thumb, and then breathe out through the left Nostril. Then repeat in similar pattern through the right nostril by closing the left. (Three times each)

2. Deeply Inhale (Left Nostril) – Exhale (Right) – Inhale (Right) – Exhale (Left) – (3 to 5 times).

You can do it three times and relax for a while observing your body. This exercise would relax you. If you find a Yoga centre, learn some physical exercise and the pranayama which is the breathing exercises. There are simple ways to keep you healthy. Instead of expensive diagnostic or treating cancer, you can perhaps lead a simple stressfree life and disease-free life which would improve your longevity. The Body is the temple, if you overutilize the senses, it will fail eventually. You need to be aware of the basics of human physiology, psychology with the behavioural analysis.

Take a good rest over the weekend. Practice these Yoga exercises, and once a year in summer travel to the nearest hill station and enjoy your life. There is no reason to feel resentment; just enjoy life to the core by leading a simple life, and be part of the Nature.

End of Session # 10

Day 10 – Session # 11:

Dr. Maddy, what is known as "SAMPATH?" and How does it impact conditioning as you had stated in one of the discussions.

Sure. I'll explain.

Formation of Habits

You'll need to understand the habits formation and the sixteen characters as indicated by Siddhas of India. These sixteen characters form the base personality.

There are factors such as Sexual Vital Fluid, Flood, Country, Education, Government, Age, Friendship, Environments, Research, Habits, Practices and Morality.

I would classify in to social and personal as the factors indicated above vary for every country, culture and every person. It is necessary to consider the behavioural science based on the above factors which forms the baseline condition:

Personality
Baseline Condition

The adulthood personality starts with the baseline condition, and then you start improving the character based on the perceptions which forms habits. For example, you are conditioned to be "GOOD" based on the set of principles taught by the RELIGION as belief based system imposed on you.

When you become an adult, You don't find it appalling. And you intend to be a REBEL which is a natural process of learning. In fact, GOD wanted ADAM and EVE to be rebellious. That's why he indicated them about the fruit of knowledge. Either you remain as a follower or rebel, learn and grow. But the message should be clear: "do not repeat the same mistake." You should learn to use the intellect reasoning as you grow.

Otherwise, you would become cyclic in your behaviour, repeating same mistakes, with results. I suggest you should learn from every mistake, and say "Thank you" for every mistake committed. It will help you grow.

Perhaps a child born in the West is not the same as in East, even a child with an Eastern origin, born in the West is transformed in a different country or vice versa. East or West, you'll need to teach your children, and help them transform the instinctively based behaviour to intuitive behaviour, without imposing 'VIRTUES' taught by the RELIGION. It is there in the SUBCONSCIOUS mind. It is your responsibility to replace it with your own "REVELATIONS" in order to comprehend TRUTH.

The need is to educate right for children, in helping them transform their consciousness. As an adult transformation process takes longer, and years to decondition, however, it is easy in childhood which should be based on the "REALIZATION BASED EDUCATION" system inculcating the right habits, regardless of country, borders as our human endeavour are to reach the fullest, blossoming in to the Nature.

The UNO has to wake up to the situation to change the World with the development of consciousness. As discussed earlier, anything done from the Outer mind without any consciousness involved would be disastrous, and you will experience the consequences at some point. The Energy of Sex transforms into love at the centre! The anger and rage will change in to magnanimity!

A paradigm shift is required from education to the politics globally. Otherwise, even Christ cannot save the world.

Dr. Maddy, please explain the power of thought.

139

The Power Of Thought

Wouldn't you understand the way of evaluation involves MIND? It is Mind as a wave trying to create a specific wavelength to retrieve a pattern from the brain cells. It is a way of replaying it from the brain. Every thought induced in mind will propel to the cosmos, and bounce back at you. A little theory of the bio-magnetic wave nature is required here. Every thought has an impact.

The Bio-magnetic Wave has five characteristics: 1) Clash, 2) Reflection, 3) Refraction, 4) Interaction and 5) Penetration and finally 6) Mind itself. As per the wave theory, thoughts are also shadow-wave, emerging from your mind will follow through the process of reflecting on a specific object which you have focused at, and then refracts back at you.

Anything that you would do or even think has a consequence as it bounces back, creating an imprint in the Genetics with a result. For example, if you clap your hands. You hear a sound. You just did an action, which is imprinted in you with a result as your experience. Just think you did not create a noise is only a transformation as you might have observed clapping your hands. The pressure you created is transformed to a noise as discussed due to the conversion of the magnetic energy. It is all manifestations of energy in myriad forms.

Zen masters call it as 'single hand clapping' which is a koan to provoke disciples to think riddles known as 'KOANS'.

Could you elaborate on Misery, Dr.?

Misery

A reference from Bhagvat Gita as advised by Krishna to Arjun, just ahead of the Kurukshetra War.

"DO YOUR DUTY WITHOUT ANTICIPATING RESULTS."

The above statement is tremendously significant and indicates the principles of '**KARMA YOGA**'. Perhaps a way of living without setting expectations, or anticipatory results? Often Misery is due to your calculations, or even hallucinate the results as you would expect. The prefixed notion in mind is the result of all miseries.

If you want to avoid your miseries, just drop expecting from every situation. Just do it, as GOD himself descending as results. If you do it right with '**IDEALISM**' as realization-based truth as per the inner revelations, you will be able to achieve uninterrupted bliss in life everywhere, in any confronting situations if your conviction of the truth is stronger.

You are responsible for all your miseries, and not anyone else. Nature tries to portray what you've got. It guides you only if you a little open. What is the point in going after temples, and churches after you have done something incorrect and expect a positive result? Nature is the '**CAUSE and EFFECT**' – what you sow is what is reaped and you cannot deny the result. Perhaps, through the way of meditation, you can sublimate it. The purpose is to be aware even before you think. Give the space in your heart a prominence before you think and act. Often the results are havoc due to the reflexive actions, instead of intuitive action in awareness, hence the miseries in mind to sum it up.

Why are we failing in love and relationships, Dr. Maddy?

Love and Relationships

Wouldn't you realize all emotions have boundaries? Just think about it. Your anger, love etc. You cannot be angry for hours

141

continuously. As you understand the science of mind, which is perceiving, as an emotion through the senses.

Mind can react through the senses or perhaps "think"; it is record and replay. It records everything as the subconscious mind and replays it from the brain cells. It is its function if you circle-back your Mind wave towards its centre; which is the conscious itself.

Tell me honestly. How many of you would concur, love and relationship is successful and happily married? It cannot sustain beyond a point, what you might be thinking as a pleasure at 20, is no more a pleasure at 40 or 50, isn't it? Your perceptions will change if you grow both biologically and spiritually. Every grey hair is an expression of truth, reminding you much closer to the self, and the Nature. Perhaps, you would have learn't the harder way. And others would have learnt through the way of books, based on experiences or through intuition. It depends on your condition, and how hard it is. At least while reading this book, you can reflect on each of these points over and over again to counsel yourself.

Now, **why are these relationships failing?** As a simple matter of fact, you are not happy within your mind as it is stagnated in mundane activities. How would you expect two stagnated minds to create happiness logically? This is exactly the problem!

A woman cannot fit a man's bill ever, due to his conditioning and the sexual desires in most of the cases. I would call it as false sensations or perhaps virtual sensations. More so, the next step after the honeymoon is over. The reality starts, when the truth begins, you'll need to have an expanded state of mind to realize your spouse as the manifestation of Nature, to sublimate your karmic-debts. You should understand the better half is the manifestation of Nature in helping you in the journey of consciousness.

It is Nature's plan to heal you, guide you and protect you from the untoward consequences, and help you transcend beyond conditioning to the ultimate consciousness itself. If you are able to comprehend to the truths, perhaps you will realize the sacrifices that she is doing to you. Women should be respected for what she is by 'Nature'. A profound transformation of a little girl, to a woman, and finally a mother where her psychology blossoms by Nature; if allowed with little efforts in meditation.

Hence, I would like to say Women are all spontaneous, and they are aligned with Nature. There is no need to think about so many conditioning. Perhaps it is a hard shell, in the minds of Men, who need to transcend negative conditioning. Only thing is that Women have the male mind (23 chromosomes). Perhaps they should be careful to stay within their Nature. Instead of thinking about expressing the male side which is not natural; their nature is feminine and Divine. There is no need to feel embarrassed being a woman. Let her be the way she is and the way Nature has designed as Mahakavi Bharti says:

'Let's burn the act of defamation to Women anywhere in the WORLD.'

Did you notice all relationships ending up in a frustration from the first love to the second love. It is all frustrating as you form a repetitive pattern in chasing women! It is not going to help. Just be yourself, and focus at the centre of the heart, practice a simplified Yoga system and love which would help you change the pattern of thinking. And then you will have the 2-Dimension. Remember, I have reserved the third dimension (3-D) as the highest peak of the consciousness!!!

Once you gain enough love within yourself, of course you should love yourself first and feel happy, and the love extends to find the right partner. If you both meditate, the male and the female minds are in the spiritual union. Perhaps the climax is revealed by the Divine Nature in the orgasmic unity of spirit in unison. Nature is looking for '**YIN**' and '**YAN**' which is the static and dynamic. It is the yearning for both the male and female minds to sublimate into the ultimate Mother. Life will be joyful ever, and you will feel the blessings, and benedictions of truth and the Leela as Krishna says. The **MAYA** or the illusion will be clear in the third dimension (3D) view to you ultimately.

Your love is made up of conditioning, and it will just last until physical layer is satisfied; The second layer is heart oriented if you are little closer the heart, it will yield thousands of poetry and art. You will be elated beyond just the physical attraction. Most of the love of the contemporary World is just the first one as you have lost the capacity to hear the music of the heart! Listen to what poet Kamba says about love:

In Ramayana, Poet Kamba says:

"The Lord looks at her beloved,
And she whispers him through her smoking eyes;
In the crescent of the balcony;

Ain't she intend to see him close,
Perhaps she did as her heart took her away,
Like a bee to the flowers;

Perhaps, like a flower to the bee,
And the bee responds looking at,
The moon's, cool shade of her forehead,
And the bow like Bro does speak;

The Lord Rama and Sita,
Both rising in Love!!!"

What A beautiful instance. Just think about the love, like a fragrance and spontaneously flowing from flower to the bees, unlike the bees chasing the flowers. The flower yielding first and the bee reckons it.

What I understood from the true love of Lord Rama and Seeta who are pure by heart following their consciousness and spontaneous with Nature.

Anything that flows out of conscious, which is termed as language of the heart is pure, and every action in the state of

144

awareness would yield blissfulness, and it cannot be the other way. If your mind is the manifestation of God, then there cannot be worries. The problem is that you work, out of the conditioned mind. And you never had a chance to expand your consciousness mind. The Universities have not explained the ways of living, and the parents have made it complicated without helping you realize the mind. Most of the spiritual leaders have condemned "sex" as against "spirituality" due to lack of understanding.

You are just one part of the cast, and the other part of the cast is somewhere in the world, which is Indeed based on the sixteen characterization; your partner has manifested to help you grow spiritually. If you are just body oriented, sooner or later you will find it irritating; you will end up in a divorce without realizing it.

If you are not truly searching from the bottom of the heart, how do you expect Nature to help! Nature conspires through the people around you, whom you meet and socialize. They reflect your conditioning. If you are not reciprocating; how would Nature talk to you?

You have closed it already, and the pores of the heart are already closed, and it is filled with mundane things. More so, in addictions your heart and lungs, becomes a scrap metal. Even the scrap metal is useful. The system becomes worse than a junk yard if you're diseased by way of excessive sexual fantasies. You have spoiled the system in acts of anger; rage etc. In temperamental moods and finally disorders in mind with conflicting thoughts, and diseases in the body, then you would be spending the whole life in treating diseases after the other.

If the life is gone, you cannot come back to this World with your own body. You have a choice to be really yourself, and enjoy moments or procastinate for nothing. It is the last chance; if you are not capable of understanding it. Then perhaps you are wasting your life. Your life will be just a fiction without any moments of benediction; Perhaps a fiction of misery, and anguish in the end of it all! You'll need to realize the benedictions offered, to the eternal life. Indeed, death is the final climax as you start the eternal journey of the spirit!!!

If you look at a woman with the above realization, wouldn't you want to thank her for the Divine Nature for her arrival at the right time and age? She is the ultimate manifestation of the Divine Nature.

Please elaborate on the Evolution; Dr. Maddy explains the Rule # 5; lineage to God

The Evolution of Nature

A simple truth is that due to the limitations of senses; all pleasures through the sensual pleasures are subjective to limitations, hence it is natural to feel limited, bored or anxiety as each of these emotions cannot get you anything more. Your inner core is hankering for more, more and more which is Nature's Instinct. Nature is eternity, with the characteristics of:

1. Super Static
2. Super Force
3. Super Consciousness

It remains as dynamic in a state, and life beings as it started manifesting itself from the absolute darkness into the elements etc.

A simple truth is that the static which is eternal and almighty, due to its self-compressive surrounding pressure force, it has broken into multiple particles known as the energy particles which started spinning in Time-T1 due to surrounding pressure force. A simple analogy is that you enclose a paper bit in to a glass bottle, and start applying pressure at all sides, the object will naturally start spinning.

1. **Step 1** – spinning action of particle derived from space, known as the energy particles.

2. **Step 2** – Since it is spinning in space, the static space media itself causing whirling shadow wave particles and the whirling shadow wave dissolves as magnetism.

3. **Step 3** – It is further manifests into elements, compounds, galaxies etc.

4. **Step 4** – Mind is the lineage of Space or super consciousness as a micro-consciousness as it evolved from a single sense to the sixth sense, which is the mind itself. Finally arrived by evolving through the single sense in plant, animals so on and so forth.

Nature has taken several million years to evolve into human consciousness. Hence, the basic instinct of consciousness is to find its own self. If the MIND is conditioned and instinctive to the external, the heart as we usually speak or the centre of the mind is micro-consciousness. This in-turn has the natural desire to merge with the centre or the ultimate consciousness.

The irony is that Nature is not enforcing anyone. If you want to remain an animal, you have chosen a path of the arduous journey without any realization, would eventually become frustrating, and in the end most of them commit suicide.

They do not see any value and in another category where the shell is a little hard, they just sink their mind in miseries and stay enclosed for life-time. But remember your inner core will forever remind you of the basic instinct of consciousness, and keep diverting it to the centre.

Your life is a constant endeavour between the 'Inner' and the Outer. A constant struggle to get back; which is the 'INNER', and the 'OUTER' and it continuously be trying to achieve its natural instinct. If you are a hard shell, perhaps due to the conditioned mind.

Your 'OUTER' is just the periphery would win the battle.

If you have a little understanding about Nature, and respect and pray, meditate; it will divert you to the INNER core which is the core of the being. Life will start with a 3-D view from the simplest of things, from playing in a sandy beach to the space journey. Finally you would be able to feel the benedictions, and blessings of the Divine Nature.

The choice is within you. Either you are the OUTER entirely or the INNER. I am not saying you should choose "either" "or". You do not need to deny either of these, just comprehend the INNER and the OUTER should follow the INNER consciousness while engaged through the senses. It is as simple as driving the vehicle, either you drive consciously or unconsciously. You know the results!

Let the light glow in each of you, let you be aware in every instance, every moment and enjoy the uninterrupted bliss there any other purpose to expanding your bank balance? It will create some additional sensual pleasures, limited emotions by boundaries. Wouldn't you believe a new car or home can give only limited happiness? It all ends within boundaries of emotions and to the limits of your sensations; only expansion of your consciousness can yield eternal bliss and the first time you would find a different meaning to your life.

A micro consciousness merging with the supreme consciousness is a start. The Outer mind would understand the inner. Perhaps well-coordinated, the journey of consciousness will appear without wasting the MIND control exclusively in the outer. You will sublimate the natural urges, and enjoy within limits in food, sex, rest and work.

What is a conflict, Dr. Maddy?

Inner Conflict

YES/NO Situation

As discussed earlier the centre of your mind is consciousness, perhaps the centre of mind is a micro-consciousness which has a Natural desire to merge with the Super Static, Super Force, Super Consciousness. Hence, there is a constant conflict between the centres of the mind which is perhaps driving you home, whilst the surface is surfing through the senses.

Just ponder:

"The centre of the mind which is driving you home, whilst the surface is surfing through the senses".

All conflicts in your mind can be resolved, if you realize the above statement. Otherwise, it will take years to realize based on the consequences as you typically bounce back every time you are in a state of despair. **"God is like a Mother"**, she would always follow her son. But, to what extent and at what expense. You are wasting the Mind power, age, consciousness, poisoning the senses, and root of sexual vital fluid etc. Perhaps at some point you cannot bounce back from the surfing of the senses as you might have already damaged the senses.

Nature is endlessly patient, beyond a point if you are hurting yourself; what can he do? You have gone too far from the shores and surfing amidst high and low tide of life; when suddenly you feel lost and fell down, you hanker to go back to the shore which does not look any nearer. You simply close your eyes and let go in surfing, and the senses will take over till the end of the spoil sport. Unfortunately, this is the pathetic state of human endeavour.

You enjoy surfing which is good, surfing through these senses, and feel the high and low. At some point, return after you study both sides and return to the shores. There is a definite need for you to go back home; otherwise you would be fully depleted, devoid of love in the heart. As the senses, will take over.

It reminds me of the Spider Man III movie; where in the villain fits in '**ROBOTIC**' arms, which are linked to his neurons. At some point, due to the malfunction, the robotic intelligent arms would start controlling him perfectly.

This is exactly true; and what is happening to each of you. You learn to use the senses, and eventually these senses take over. For example, overeating over a period of time, resulting in diabetes or over thinking, and excessive indulgence in sexual misconduct. This result in causing a number of sexually transmitted diseases, so on and so forth;

You got to understand the mind power is wasted through these senses, causing all disaster. Perhaps the inner wants eternity; while the outer conditioning expects some sensual pleasures which are based on the natural urges. These two aspects of mind are in constant confrontation, leaving you in a schizophrenic split.

You have to understand the basic conditioning, the natural urge of the body and the infinite urge of the consciousness. The instinctive urge of consciousness is the supreme knowledge to reach back to the ocean of infinite consciousness. Unless you fulfil this need, whatever you do through the senses cannot yield any happiness. Instead, it will lead to over sensual pleasures exploiting your body, mind. Thus, resulting in pain and diseases and all sorts of mental disorder.

Instincts

Soul-Unite with Infinite

Mind-Unite with Li Mind

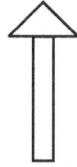

Body Urge (Basic Instincts)

Each of it has its own boundaries of emotions, when you are body oriented. You will listen to the basic urges and not transcend beyond. If you are mind oriented, a little more awareness would yield the love, with the basic instincts of the body solved. Though you start with the body, you should grow vertically upwards towards spirit.

The science of yoga is to centre you towards the consciousness, which is intended to circle-back mind towards its own centre. If the mind is an excited state say in Beta state of mind, which is the emotional state, there is no way you would comprehend truths. You will just give way to the conditioning and the pattern of wave based on the animal instincts; hence, your senses would develop a semi-conscious to take over. This will be a dangerous situation, like giving away your car keys to a stranger. Your condition is like a monkey, which keeps straying.

Once you start focusing your mind, and practice meditation to reduce the wavelength. The conditioning will subsidize eventually leaving your mini-mind to circle back and aligned with the consciousness. This correct alignment is called 'ENLIGHTENMENT', which is the ultimate journey of consciousness.

You should try and align yourself as you have been straying in the Mind for years now, and centuries through the conditioning inherited, perhaps thousands of years, due to the animal instincts.

God has provided the ability to recover from the conditioning which is the external state; realize, enjoy within limits through senses and transcend. This is intelligence, the one who is capable of realizing by analyzing the experience, the current situation and future results based on the 'CAUSE andEFFECT' theory. In simple terms, conflicts are due to the violation to the laws of Nature's **CAUSE and EFFECT**; if you think against Nature, it will happen with its consequences of pain, anguish.

You keep talking about MIND RADAR, What is it, Dr. Maddy?

Mind Radar

What you perceive through the senses in one thing, what you believe is different. Perhaps your Mind is functioning as radar, as indicated below:

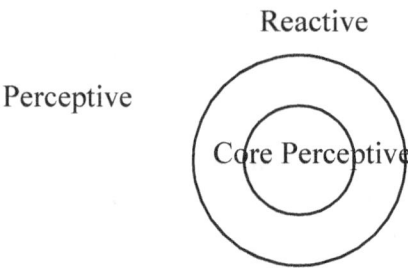

1) **REACTIVE:** Reacting quickly at the surface as a reactive MIND; When you are reactive, you are action on the reflex; based on the reactive action responding to the circumstantial stimuli.

2) **PERCEPTIVE:** Perceptive based on the reality and acceptance of results with cognitive intelligence;

   A little more awareness into perceptive mind would help you realize based on your analysis. You do not affix results in your mind; you would anticipate and acceptance of results as it is without a prefixed notion in Mind.

3) B– Centre of Consciousness itself;

   The final CORE is the centre itself where you respond, rather not react based on the consciousness itself.

I have heard, '**ZEN MONASTERY – EAST AND WEST**'

There were two Zen monasteries right opposite to each other, one facing East and the other one facing the West.

Zenko, who belongs to the East and his master advised him not to talk to the West side disciples.

Zenko, listen, '**Do not talk to these guys opposite to you; they will confuse you as they are not real yogis. Bogis indeed, they do nothing.**'

Zenko: "Ok, master."

The other disciple was instructed exactly the same.

Master: Zenko: Wesky does not talk to them as they claim to be Yogis doing nothing.

"Ok. Master!!!" Wesky responded.

Zenko walks up the hill to get some flowers for the Morning Prayer, everyday in the morning.

Wesky walks up to fetch water, chop wood!

Zenko asks, 'where are you going dude?'

Wesky replies, 'I am going wherever my leg takes.'

A little amused he goes back to his master discussing the response.

Master: I told you, they will confuse you, provoke you to the outer.

Tell them what if your leg takes you to the fire.

The next morning he tells them the same thing.

Wesky: "I will catch the fire for the cooking morning soup for my master and asks where are you going?"

Zenko: I'm going to the temple for prayer.

Wesky: To do what?

Zenko: To pray, meditate. How do you pray?

Wesky: I don't pray.

Zenko: Is it? Really, never heard of a disciple not praying. Then what do you do from the day till evening?

Wesky: "By chopping wood for cooking food, and fetching water from the well."

Zenko: Is that all you do? with a big laugh!

Wesky: "Of course."

Both of them decide to learn each other's way of living and they plan for a place up the hill to learn each other's way.

After a while, both monastery's head's meet up and discuss:

East Head: "How are you?"

West Head: "I am fine, thank you."

"Did you see your boys coming this side?"

"Of course, I do. Each of them, as we planned to both these ways; now. Our problems are resolved. Let them go to the World."

A beautiful story. The above story of Zenko and Wesky indicates your inner and the outer. You cannot ignore neither of these as a matter of fact. God wants you to know both, and transcend the senses, by limited enjoyment and awareness. When you are ready to receive the pure consciousness, it will explode into itself, and no need to force anything.

Saint and Siddha, Maharishi Vethathiri has said,

"There is no need to torture your body for spirituality,

Body is the temple of God".

You have to balance between the INNER and the OUTER. Perhaps a little more awareness when you equip your senses, through the mind. This would help you transcend eventually to the next plane of life to achieving the third dimension (3-D) in life.

Please explain the Sixth Sense, Dr. Maddy.

End of Session # 11

Day 11 – Session # 12:

Let's examine the ultimate Sixth Sense. Martin, what is the sixth sense?

Perhaps, Brain!

"Well. That's partially correct."

"Let me explain, Martin. The five sensations are pressure, sound, ligth, smell and taste. Hence, Nature has endowed you with the sense-organs to perceive sensations through the respective senses. You have five sense-organs: ear, nose, toungue, eyes, skin and the ultimate sixth sense is Mind, which is a magnetic circuit or 'wave' that can play back its sensations via brain cells. The brain cell is just a mechanism to store and retrieve like a hard disc of a computer. It can store Terrabytes (TB) of data and has the ability to connect to the Cloud network, which is the Eternal consciousness."

The SIXTH SENSE

Do you realize MIND is WAVE and measured in wavelength in cycles per second (CPS)?

Mental Frequency

As we discussed, Mind is a WAVE and frequency are measured in BETA, ALPHA, THETA and DELTA. The mental frequency is measured in cycles per second (cps) as indicated below:

     1. Beta (14-40 cps)
     2. Alpha (7-13 cps)
     3. Theta (3-6 cps)
     4. Delta (0.5-2 cps)

The lower the frequency, closer you get to GOD. In other words, GOD is the Zeroth state, and the nearest possibility is Delta (0.5-2 CPS) state of mind with revelations of truth. Most of you are in the Beta and Alpha which is the extension of the mind in thoughts, and sensual pleasures. The MIND wave cannot reach the subtle state of Mind in Theta or Delta due to the conditioning; and the past karmic-debts. Through constant practices and sublimation techniques, you can reach the Divine Nature by attuning your MIND WAVE to the super-consciousness.

Now, it is clear each of you can practice the attunement. You will be able to research any topic, build a skill to attune on a particular subject, and Nature will help you in subsequent steps. It is not philosophy, rather it is science, by way of the wave nature. I would say GOD is a democrat, as there is no difference in the way you'll feel love of the Divine Nature. All copyrights and Intellectual Property are common for all. It may be one Einstein or Mahatma, but it is due to the collective consciousness.

We respect scientists for the efforts, intelligence and perseverance. But the irony is that it is due to Nature's act of collective consciousness, and support it has originated from that point of source. No one can stop time, which is in a continuum, and why do you make an enormous fuss about the past instances. Perhaps a paradigm shift is required to allow each of you to evolve through the expanding consciousness. There is no point in accumulating the University degree without realizing self, and its lineage to Nature.

All these emotions have limits, if you do not understand the limitations of senses, you are wasting time. Perhaps east and West have to unite to formulate an education system for the mankind, thereby teaching values of the **BODY-MIND, and SPIRIT**. Sigmund Freud has introduced the behavioural science in the WEST, and the saints of EAST have attained Enlightenment. These are true assets, that you should leverage to benefit the mankind. Perhaps parents should be educated with the behavioural analysis of children, and help them get out of the conditioning through Western analysis, combined with the Eastern mythology in practices. There is none called unintelligent or perhaps a sinner. It is all your religion and priests who have condemned people. Christ said:

'Oh lord pardon their sins. Help them achieve immortal peace as they do not realize what they have done.'

Bless thy soul,
Thou, shall be forgiven,
In the kingdom of God,
For all the mistakes,
In lack of awareness;

Perhaps those who have interpreted Bible had politicized, "SIN" is government. Only awareness is the real religiousness of Buddhas, Christs and Vethathiri. They had never condemned anyone except politics!

In my view, people are just reactive that's all, based on the conditioning and the characterization. In any situation, an individual alone is not responsible. If there is violence in the US, think about the high school shooting incidences, and relate it to the violent WWF TV shows, and the violent games and consoles which is conditioning at the root. Your children are accumulating so many things, and how will they throw the conditioning out? **"WWF and any other violent mobile gaming will manifest as actions in the adult age."**

In similar terms, children are exposed to movies of crime, violence against women which is the cause of crime against women everywhere. These children hid their emotions, repress in the name of 'RELIGION', without even realizing the basics of sexual vital fluid and the differences in the male/female anatomy; this is the cause of all pornography, due to repressions. It ultimately ends up poisoning the sexual vital fluid which is the source of life.

A little awareness in each of these topics would help, and it is easy for the schools all over the World to implement. I believe Nation such as the United States can implement it in no-time.

Nature is democracy; hence we should come up with World Wide Education (WWE) with the support of United Nation Organization (UNO) implementing simple procedure to change the process of thinking.

The feelings and emotions of the heart centre are perfectly stagnated in the current way of education since there is more emphasis in the analysis through 'head', we should take the best practices of the modern education. Combine our ancient school of wisdom and meditation to realize the values.

Dr. Richard, could you explain the lineage to GOD?

"First of all, if you want to analyze GOD, you should get rid of the concept of your hell and heaven, and drop your perceptions of GOD as someone sitting a top in heavens."

There is no one there as our Scientists have ventured into the Moon and Mars. These are ways to inculcate a moral behaviour. Even my 5 years old kid won't believe it now in this mobile-age technology. Perhaps your religion is over a thousand years old and outdated in many aspect in rituals. The hidden truth has been lost due to rituals, as you're holding on to the rituals without realizing the underlying values of truth.'

"Ok. Dr. I agree. Please teach me the Scientific revelations of GOD theory."

Let's understand science little bit and then will help you understand the lineage to GOD. Every object in the Universe is made up of atoms and further if you analyze, it is made up of protons, neutrons etc. This is Science.

The Eastern Sages and Siddhas have gone a step ahead in analyzing the fundamental particle, which is known as the Energy Particle.

"Oh, is it Dr.?"

"Yes. These Scientists have had these concepts revelated by Nature as inner revelations of truth in the absolute state of meditativeness."

"Interesting Dr."

"We should thank them for their revelations and analyze it scientifically to find holistic truth in everything."

"Of course."

Einstein has explained the SPACE theory. SPACE-TIME as a continuum. The saints of the East have had the revelations of SPACE in the meditative state. They have indicated SPACE as the surrounding pressure force, and its manifestations of myriads of energy.

Rule # 5 - Realize Mind, And Lineage To Eternity

When the static became dynamic, energy particles had formed as wave due to the surround pressure force. First you need to understand the Nature, to be able to appreciate the evolutionary process and your lineage of truth. 'GOD is SPACE'. The static with the qualities of 1) Force and 2) Consciousness; the force is further classified into a) Centripetal and b) Centrifugal forces.

It is almighty self-compressive surrounding pressure force; which is excited at some point turning static into dynamic, due to this significant expansion of itself causing whirling wave particle, known as the 'Energy Particles' which are high spinning particles.

A simple analogy is that wave, and the ocean. Wave is a fraction of the Ocean, isn't it? In a similar context, the Divine Fluid with its self-compressive Nature manifested into fraction, and started whirling with high velocity due to its surrounding pressure force. This is the first particle, which is the energy particle. The supreme consciousness has four factors: **1) Force, 2) Time, 3) Volume and 4) Distance**.

Each of these particles creates ripple waves due to its whirling motion; it creates a ripple in the media of the Divine Natural field, thereby causing ripple waves or the shadow wave particles, which eventually dissolves into the media itself as '**MAGNETISM**'. This is known as the Universal Secret in ancient days, in India. Now the energy particles have grouped to form atom, what scientists claim, and elements, compounds till the **Galaxies and Universes bound by the law of Nature.** Nature has evolved with a physical structure in the human beings, with five senses of pressure, sound, light, smell and taste. The organs were formed based on these five conversions, with the reproductive organs. These imprints are coded as cumulative imprints in the form of Genetics and transferred to the progeny as characterization. **The final sixth-sense has evolved with an ability to identify the secrets of Nature through surrender and love.** It's like wave and the ocean as Bhagvat Gita says. The analogy here is that wave is mind, whilst the ocean is the pure consciousness or GOD.

Finally, the climax is that humans have evolved with all cumulative experiences, characterization in genetics, with an additional sense, known as the '**SIXTH SENSE**', which is the ultimate sense in the evolution of **Nature to Man**? The sixth sense is capable of perceiving things with its revelations of Nature, which is your ultimate '**MIND**'.

As Einstein has highlighted 'SPACE, TIME, VOLUME and FORCE are in continuum. In other words, there is a media on which the whole Universe is floating in the SKY in the dark Divine fluid. The gravitational force was initially perceived by Newton as force from the object. For example, an apple falling down from the tree is due to the gravitation pull of Earth. However, this concept was not complete. Einstein revealed the SPACE, TIME, VOLUME and FORCE as continuum. This indcates there is a media on which the Universe is floating. However, Einstein was not clear how on where the force is generated within energy particles. The saint, Vethathiri of our times has demonstrated the 'UNIFIED FORCE' theory, where the reason for the enormous force generated in the energy particles is due to the surrounding pressure force, which is the ultimate STATIC and DIVINE fluid, known as the 'UNIFIED FORCE' by the Scientists, and 'GOD' by the Spiritualist.

The human physiology is a replica of the Universe with the centre of MIND as consciousness. The life-force particles are whirling causing ripple waves in the Divine Fluid, thereby causing countless thousands of wave generated which is the '**MIND**'. It further dissolves through the senses as sensations and Mind perceives and restores it as enjoyment.

Nature has taken millions of years to evolve into what you are now, from the static to dynamic, and inanimate to the animate. Theron, it has evolved its senses from a single sense, plant to the sixth sense as the '**MIND WAVE**'. A beautiful body, mind and soul feeling the sensations of pain, pleasure, peace; Your personality is the cumulative experiences of mind. You'll need to evaluate that from time to time, without being subjected to the emotional state as each of these karmic debts can lead you to misery.

Cumulative Experiences of Mind

The understanding of mind is necessary. It is essential to understand the manifestations of Nature, with the available tool called 'MIND'; which is a bio-computer. I was contemplating about Mind's functions and sensations, analyzing various facets of Mind's functions; here is an excerpt and a fascinating analogy:

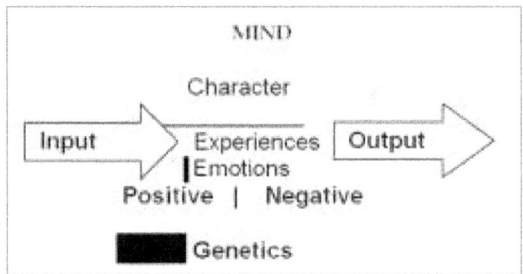

MIND is conditioned as we already discussed. You have to understand the functions and its behaviour a little closely. Pay attention.

1. Character
2. Experiences
3. Emotions
4. Positive
5. Negative

These are the three primary functions as it evaluates every situation based on your conditions, and the condition is based on the baseline genetics, and cumulative experiences are known as the (a) 'Prarabhda Karma / Sanchita Karma' and the (b) 'Acamiya Karma'; each of these past and present karmic debts accumulated in you till date. The past karma is due to the heriditary, and the present karma is due to your own actions. You don't need to be startled by the facts as you've a way to sublimate karmic debts. There are profound techniques from the ancient Yogic practices such as the progressive and regressive therapy techniques that will help you sublimate. These practices combined with the Psychiatry will help you in healing the conditioning.

Now, the point here is to analyze a specific situation and realize how you would reach as output causing action. Indeed, this is a wonder as I realized its conditioning, and its function,as a result, causing your core personality, and characterization in evaluating through the sense. This is virtually playing back the past events in memory to correct the sequences, the genetic sequence will be decoded. I've heard about a legendary cricketer, Sachin Tendulkar who use to watch his past videos to motivate himself. This is a way of regressive analysis. Think about the success stories in your life to gain inner strength, or the failures that would have improved your endurance. You are much stronger now. These cumulative actions will become your personality as a result.

Let's analyze your past events inflicting pain in you. Anyone such event of significance in your life:

A painful and traumatic experience; let's analyze it, and be aware; I am going to take you through the trauma again. But this time you will be aware of the drama in the stage of mind, hence do not subject yourself to the painful emotions. Think about the trauma of an emotional distress and pain that you felt the last time when you were suffering from post-operative traumatic experiences, or a broken relationship. You have a laundry list, perhaps.

The above traumatic experiences will yield two types of emotion; one is that you have gone through the agony first which are the painful sensations; now the right stuff, as it always comes after the pain, as all happiness does! The richest was poorest someday, and the oldest was the youngest some day, and so on and so forth.

The healthy stuff is the character, your conviction and 'WILL' power that had gotten you past the situation with your character and ability to succeed the moment itself. Did you realize the point? Of course, you did go through the traumatic experiences as painful sensations; and it lasted for a while where you were victimized. Alright; the rightstuff followed then, and you came out of the situation say. For example, Your addictions to the alcohol, anger, or immoral passion etc. Now, you feel stronger than before, and perhaps, like a Robert Bruce who had succeeded.

Have you heard this?

Robert Bruce said 'My success is based on the 99 failures.'

It is true Indeed, as you may exclaim.

You have come out of the traumatic experiences based on the WILL and character that you have the ability to transform depressive state of MIND to an expression, and you did well in the past doing so.

Now, You have realized your trauma, and the inherent ability of your MIND coming out in style. You think about these experiences and realize that you could have averted the situation. By expanding the consciousness and the MIND's capacity to transform temperamental behaviour. The final step in the above experience, what have you gained. You have added more strength to the character, isn't it?

Now, you will comprehend the inherent Nature and capacity of the mind expanding and resolve all conflicts. The intelligence is there, and you need to uncover the truth. That's all. Perhaps you will need a little effort to analyze these experiences, and analyze the positive emotions; which is realizing your ability to transform a situation and come out of it.

Based on the cumulative experiences, hold on firmly to the 'sensations of positive emotions' and how much you cherished coming out of the traumatic experiences and how much you felt energized and successful. I believe you have gone through the above instance in multiple occasions; the only issue is that you have been hanging on to the traumatic experiences it, instead of hanging on to the experiences of how you succeeded in coming out of it.

This is what Nature wants you to learn through MIND, which can record and replay as you need. The inherent capacity is to introspect; every situation to transform ordinary circumstances, into extraordinary circumstances, and the painful emotions as the path to the paradox of bliss, and ecstasy.

The above phenomena are your experience. Just think about it. The success you have had in getting over an addictive state of mind or perhaps the experience of succeeding over a trauma. **How much courageous you were?** Isn't that your character, and core personality? Hang on to it, to the character of strength and the answers coming from within you. Do you think the last time when you were in a need, you got the help? Just think about it, the background story is that.

God or the **DIVINE** Fluid or the cosmic consciousness has helped you through someone. Perhaps, pain is an occasion where you have derailed yourself from the Natural laws where you have flaunted by the wrong doing, hence the pain. It is not God's intention. It was your action and GOD's result. This is what highlighted in Bhagvat Gita.

"I'll reveal myself in everything."

It indicates GOD manifesting as result of your actions. When a ball hits the ground, it bounces back, and the intensity of it depends on how much you have thrown. Perhaps you threw a conflicting thought, resulting in action which is propelling at you as pain!

It was your action, and God is the result, it was not his fault, and it was your ignorance. The past reaction is gone, and now you are in a Time which is in the continuum. There is no need to repent, or feel disguised about the past. Now, you are stronger than before as the situation has taken you to the core of your being and rattled it. Well.

Here is my approach:

"Be Aware of the sensations, and research without being subjected to the sensitivity."

Have you observed a night watchman who is constantly aware all night? Or perhaps like an emotional movie, where you see people fighting, and you are just watching. Just watch the movie inside the mind.

165

Think about the traumatic experiences. Be an observer; perhaps take five (5) deep breaths to view it through the consciousness, not through the senses. You will realize how stupid you were. Subjected to the emotions that do not exist.

'**MIND IS WAVE**' then emotions are shadow wave that does not exist, and you are holding on to the flux; Be aware and centered, when your senses excite you. There is no reason to feel antagonistic against the negative emotions, as these emotions in a way shown the way to heaven. I've heard a chinese proverb: '**If you know the way to hell, then the way to heaven is a lot easier**'.

Now, you are stronger than ever, but the only fact is that avoiding repeating mistakes in the cyclic pattern due to addictions. You should be aware through the introspective and meditative practices to sublimate it and transcend tracing the source of the negative emotions. You are lucky; perhaps you have gone through these emotions.

At least you have had the opportunity to transcend when compared to those dead-sanyas over the Himalayas. There is no need for sanyas in Himalayas, there is no one to excite their mind, perhaps it is their comfort to feel. All those upside –down techniques are not going to help you at all to transcending your emotions.

You need a psychological analysis, to uproot your emotions, sensations to go to the root, and transform it. Perhaps a little Freud's theory would help in behavioural analysis. And do not forget to say thank you '**MY DEAR EMOTIONS**', you have helped me transform and transcend beyond. It is my experience as well as you would get stronger. All these negative emotions will help you transcend towards eternity, and reach the peak of consciousness.

Only fact is that you should come out of the cyclic pattern, do it with a little more awareness. If you miss the point, then try it again. Reflect on your thoughts. Nature is expecting you to be receptive by opening the heart towards realization. Nature will conspire to find the right contacts for you to reach the Divine. After all this is all Shakespearean play, where you are a cast to demonstrate on the stage; if you realize the film that is constantly projecting on your MIND, it will reveal the emotions.

As a matter of fact in business, there is a newer trend in most of the corporates are trying to identify the managers, those who have gone through the crisis situations. The one who has transformed crisis to an opportunity is the 'most wanted' manager. In a similar analogy, I would say a man who has gone through the variety of emotions; traumatized, tortured is the one who would realize it easily'.

Mind is a friend, and the only tool available to reach the Divine; hence, treat him with all due respect, and align it to your consciousness. If you practice a simple breathing technique; you will become aware of the senses, which can transform it to spiritual experiences.

Dr. Richard continued to explain intense ways of memory technique.

Memory Technique

Memorizing is something that you are trying to store in mind; it is rather easier than you think. For example, if you want to memorize a specific term, you have to reduce the mental frequency, and store it as a strand in the brain cells; In cases of your failure to recollect which is due to the inability of mind to attune to a particular wavelength. Mind is a bio-magnetic wave, and it stores everything it observes into the brain cells, genetics and the sensing organs. Hence, you need to be practicing your MIND to attune to a specific wavelength.

For example, if you are studying about **E=MC²**, Einstein's Electron wave Nature, you need to be in a subtle wavelength in order grasp the subject. Whenever you want to replay from memory, you'll need to go to the subtle state as recorded. At times, you were unable to recollect, which indicate you are excited, without being able to reach the subtle state of mind.

Whenever you're filled with the bio-magnetic energy, the conditioning will start surfacing. If you are a little aware, perhaps you can guide it safely to the beneficial activities by using the mind power positively. Also, progress towards spiritually by analyzing your deeper instincts, as it will need a lot of energy within.

Instead, if you are just relying on the temporary solution, then your thoughts will escalate when you are silent. And it will play the spoil sport. Hence, most of you are afraid to be alone just staying alone in silence. Try to be silent for a day, contemplate which would take you to the deeper insights itself.

Anecdote: Adam and Eve

God created Adam and Eve in the Garden of Eden, they were much uncivilized asking for everything to God for help.

Well. God thought within himself and planned drama to play. He said:

"Ok. Adam and Eve there is a tree out there and do not eat the 'apple' fruit of the tree", but you have everything you would like beautiful glaciers. Perhaps to their amusement Adam and Eve, kept looking at the tree, got closer and never tried to eat.

She plucked the fruit from the tree in all her embarrassment, to find what it is in there.

"Oh my God!" Adam said.

God witnessed it, Well. Nothing as Adam said trying to save Eve from her mistake. This is the first instance of his own personality, 'lying' to God and dishonesty. Finally, they both were expelled from the Garden of Eden.

This is a beautiful story. I believe the idea is subjective as God himself conspired ADAM to rebel and experience everything to return to heaven. Otherwise what is the use of the senses! Perhaps, a little awareness could have transformed Adam and Eve to the temple of consciousness back to the Garden of Eden. Perhaps the fruit of knowledge has been given to you, and the entire life is a journey towards realizing it. Your intrinsic values, you have been expelled from the Garden of Eden, several times. Alright. Fine. Move on and identify the conditioning and transcend.

You are stronger than before; the instances of pain, miseries, anguish, fear and anxiety have made you stronger and the strongest perhaps. You were not sitting with closed eyes in Himalayas, which is good for cowards. Perhaps you are a newer breed of human consciousness. You have realized the pains and beyond.

The only quest is to realize the character that you have gained over the ordeals, and do not repeat it over and over again. Otherwise, you would form a cyclic pattern holding on to the pattern, instead of the truth. My request to each of you is that, try to analyze the character that you have gained by succeeding in a painful endeavour. This would strengthen further and further. Enough of these painful instances, and sufferings get over your conditioning and visualize your strong character and the centre '**CONSCIOUSNESS**' that has helped you at every instance whenever you sought help.

I request you to hold on to the '**CHARACTER**' the ultimate character of strength, and the values that you carry at the centre and move on from the past conditioning. There is no need to be antagonistic with your mind, and its behavioural pattern of sex, anger. Which are all the manifestations of the same energy in a state of flux? Perhaps a little understanding and the awareness would help you transcend from the cyclic pattern.

Anecdote for you

A disciple arrived at the monastery. When Buddha was on his regular alms '**BoudhiBichshanthi**' asking for alms in the neighborhood.

One of his prime disciple interacted this new man and asked "What do you want?"

Man: "Oh Master, teach me meditation."

Ananda: "Our master is out. Let me check."

He walked to the monastery to find the disciple of Buddha, who is an expert in astrology.

Haiku: "Well. Let me read your past conditioning, he exclaimed oh no."

Ananda: "What happened Haiku?" This man has had the worst history in the current and the past lives. He has been a murderer, rapist, etc. And never had followed a single virtue.

Haiku: "Ok. I will send him out. Man, we have decided not to initiate you in to the monastery." Please go before Buddha comes here in few minutes.

Man: "Oh no Sir. I need meditation. I would follow it; Master, please teach me meditation."

"Ok." He waited at the door step for Buddha, the enlightened master. Buddha arrived with intense vibrations, and valor of a thousand elephants. He found it like a soft white light embracing him…and prostrate under his feet.

"Oh my beloved Master, 'help me'."

"**I know,** he was a famous murderer in town."

Buddha was referring to all his past conditioning, looking deep through his eyes, and he walked in silently asking him to come in.

170

Both Ananda and Haiku were a little surprised.

"Oh master, I read his astrology and found his past **KARMAS**. This man can never meditate, not even for a single split second." Buddha smiled gently and said, perhaps, he is the ideal candidate. And proceed towards initiating him into the monastery.

After a few months. The man was joyously singing, dancing and whirling.

Ananda and Haiku: "Master, did you see him? He is disturbing our meditation and the disciples here in the monastery."

Buddha said, 'Just let him go. And leave him alone.'

I name him Dharma as he has achieved enlightenment this morning. When I met him with the eyes filled with grace and the melting emotions of the past conditioning. He has achieved, through intensive practices and the pains, miseries, anguish, sufferings that he has had in the past six lives, have transformed him. Just a glimpse of truth has helped in realize it totally.

What a beautiful story?

Did you reflect on the conditioning?

Just move on, if you are reading this, close your eyes and let the emotions melt away entirely. Christ, Buddha and Bodhi Dharma, Saint and Vethathiri are all awaiting you to open the heart a little more and pay attention to these emotions. It is the society responsible for the plight.

Perhaps you have learnt it now, and the personality can be shifted in the magic quadrant and your consciousness can be elevated. As a witness, I see you picked up this book to analyze your past conditioning, and emotions which is a beginning. This is the beginning of your evolving consciousness, and the truth will reveal. This will be your inner revelations, which you would teach to your children, and millions of children in Africa, Pakistan as the entire World would shrink to a Global

Village. A village of oneness singing hymns of truth, and music composed in consciousness.

Sing, Dance and Rejoice

Let the singing begin,
Let the dance begin,
The spirit yearns to grow;
As it is eternal and
Natural!

The consciousness is the centre;
Perhaps a state of flux,
A little overdoes of flux,
In a state of slumber!

Good. You have realized!
My dear brothers and sisters,
Let the consciousness evolve,
Let the consciousness grow,
Let the consciousness reveals,
The secrets of Nature!

Let alone the consciousness become,
Part of the eternal truth!

Let you not be there as senses;
Let you not be there as Ego;

Let you sing, dance and rejoice;
In the blossoming consciousness,
To the fullest!

The story of Supreme to the minuscule,
Back to the Supreme!!!!

Before wrapping up the session Dr. Richard, Martin and Dr. Maddy, invites a few other professors on stage...

Martin continues...

Dear All, These days that I have spent at Dr. Richard's office of Mental Health with his profound wisdom, and subsequent discussions with Dr. Maddy has helped me gain confidence, to realize my spiritual being.

Plan for some quality time! It is pathetic to see a large number of diseases due to the hectic phase of life in the name of Globalization! We remorse for the lost life, and lost happiness due to the hectic pace of life; there is a larger problem which is killing in the sedentary life-style in the commercialization of time. Life has become a commodity. You go through it, and there is no plan to enjoy the moments.

End of Session # 12

Day 12 – Session # 13:

Practice Awareness

Dr. Maddy and Richard continue to explain the methods to practicing awareness!!!

I would like to start off with an anecdote.

Anecdote for you to start with

A Zen monk, Wei Hung asked one of his disciples about the virtues of life.

The disciple wrote something, and he returned to the master after ten minutes.

Ah...Honu; "Do not come to me with this, go to the University to learn the virtues of life."

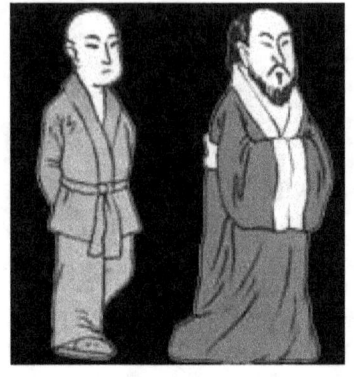 Honu was a bit amused, and he returned back after a week and said, "Master, I have studied the virtues of life now after spending years in the University, and corrected it by discussing it with the eminent professors etc. And a beautiful write-up as a result," Honu was showcasing his credentials to claim recognition for his work!

"Alright. Meet Wu Li - Go to the distant village and learn the art from the master."

Honulu was even more amused as he had to travel over a thousand miles to a distant village to meet Wu Li, a Zen master.

Wu Li responded when asked about the Virtues in life:

"Before enlightenment chop wood and carry water.
After enlightenment, chop wood and carry water."

- Wu Li

And he continued to fetch water from the well.

Finally Honulu arrives back, and he was almost about to lose his control as he felt betrayed and outrageous.

Wei Hung says: "Well Honulu; It cannot be studied in a University, nor any book can teach you."

"You can practice it right now in the moment to moment awareness."

Awareness is a state of the subtle mind, acting through consciousness. The centre is the lead, with the surface following the centre. You'll be able to achieve only if you've sublimated the karmic debts. Otherwise your consciousness will be clouded by the dust of karma's like a mirror clouded in dust.

AWARE – Get over the temperamental Moods

Setup your **IDEALISM** through the inner revelations of Truth. If you are aware, actions-results and karmic influences will all be in sync with the universal laws.

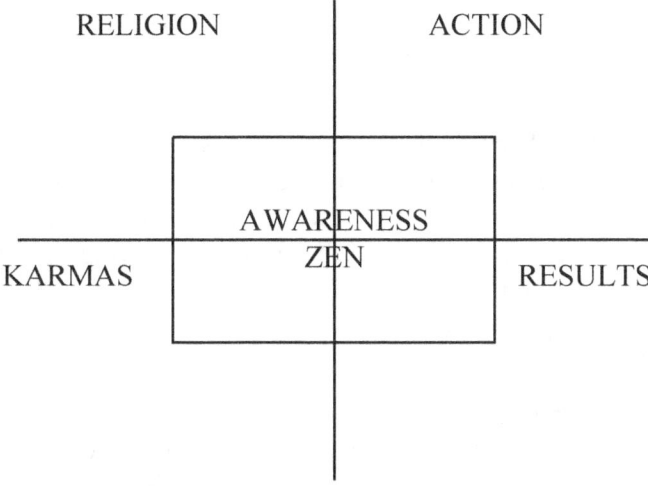

Be aware of your thoughts, if you would like to succeed. These thoughts are treasures, which will teach you something and realize it for expanding it to the super consciousness.

As you practice, you will find changes in behaviour. Just write down changes weekly and every change that you would like to achieve over a period of time. You can visualize your personality after a year (s) spiritually grown personality, blossoming in Nature.

All I am saying is that to prioritize your well being ahead of anything else. Your inherent Nature is eternity. It is like an 'Internet' connecting you to the larger network called GOD.

As you've realized meditation is one half of the story, that will help you regain and conserve energy. However, the other half is introspection to sublimate the karmic debts by the way of analysis.

Dr. Please explain Meditation and Introspective Analysis.

Meditation and Introspective Analysis

As discussed, Meditation is not an endeavour of twenty minutes, and it is not contemplating on something. It is an absolute dissolution of self into the super consciousness. It is the ultimate reunion of the micro consciousness with the macro consciousness.

The process of meditation is often misunderstood by a lot of people as concentration; which is not true. You start of focusing attention on chakras, then you will start sublimating thoughts. Once you align mind properly through by lowering the mental frequency (wavelength), will lead you to the thoughtless state of mind which is known as '**NO MIND**'.

You're using the '**MIND**' to focus, reduce its wavelength. And eventually you merge with the cosmos. If you can extend this state of '**NO MIND**' everywhere in any occasion, your life will be blissful. And you'll be able to access the three dimensional (3-D) views of life.

When you start meditating, thoughts will distract initially. By and by it will subdue as you would focus on centering on chakras's then alignment of MIND with cosmos would yield life as a benediction. The art of meditation to circle back from outer to inner; by focusing your attention from senses to the consciousness itself which is the source of it.

Martin, I am going to teach you a simple and profound technique that you can follow. You can practise this exercise anywhere!

Now, let us analyze the evolutionary process of mind and your ability to traverse back to the past events.

Let the BODY, MIND and SPIRIT be healed. You are feeling light, lighter and lightest.

You are eternal! Drop your name, identify that was created by the society, and merge with the pure consciousness, just like a dew drop merging into an Ocean; you are now part of the supreme consciousness and just float in this cosmic energy for some time. There is no time here and not even dynamics of force, as you are in the absolute space. If you want to go trance, go-ahead and enjoy swimming in the cosmic ocean; let it guide you and stay there for a while. You are as pure as a rose flower! Just smell the divinity in you, a perfume, a Divine perfume in the body.

There is nothing in mind as you have lost the past conditioning, baggage that you have been carrying. Just laugh how untrue it was, and the illusion that burst a while ago! The emotional bubble has just burst, and the heart is open like a lotus flower in the wilderness into eternity; you are listening to the songs of the birds and you are enjoying the moments of bliss.

Observe human beings, birds, and the pet dog by focusing at the heart centre. You can counsel in the expanded state of mind. Perhaps you can talk to the Divine right now through the heart! The inventions of the WEST belong to the EAST, and the intuition of the EAST belongs to the WEST. Indeed both are synonyms to the OUTER and the INNER mind. Whilst East is INNER and WEST is the Outer. The modern man will be balanced between the two; he will be able to transcend through his conditioning by analyzing the behaviour sciences.

The following technique progressive and regressive therapy will heal your past conditioning. Martin, you'll need to practice this exercise on a regular basis.

Rule # 6 Practice Awareness

Progressive and Regressive Evolution

Your mind has evolved through the progressive evolution of Nature itself from the single sense plant to the sixth sense, which is mind. Did you know you have the ability to retrospect regressively? Meaning, you can go back to the past events. This indicates traversing back in time to identify the past imprints, and rectify it. Alternatively, in the progressive evolution of mind, you will be able to analyze the future consequences of any action. In regressive evolution, you have the ability to correct the past experiences of trauma and psychic disorders.

This will help in psychiatric treatment in treating disorders, addictions. For example, the '**PROGRESSIVE**' evolution technique to analyze the situation in the future. The '**REGRESSIVE**' evolution technique will involve projections of the past situation; This is one of the therapy patient will follow through the experiences as an observer, rather than being subjective to the situation.

The Bhagvat Gita introduces the karma Yoga as the way of indifference, without submerging into the worldly pleasures. You should be like a lotus flower on water. How will you achieve without a practice by analyzing your inner self? Once your conditioning is removed, you'll reflect the pure consciousness.

Introspection is a way of contemplating on the conditioning as you have to use the 'MIND'as a tool for external activities, by engaging relevant senses. If you are aware while engaging the senses, you will know the limits. If you are not aware, then you will exceed limits causing pain.

After the daily meditation, you might have observed its frequency lowering in a subtle state of mind; hence you become aware of its conditioning at a higher frequency. You can use one of the profound methods such as a mind-mapping technique to identify the conditioning and transcend.

Both meditation and introspection will complement each other. Also, you are now aware of the six temperamental moods, human behavioural science and simple and profound therapies available to you to transcend.

Try a simple breathing technique.

Simple physical exercise and then,

Meditate by focusing on chakras meditation A.K. Agnichakra, which is between the eyebrows if you're initiated. For rest, follow the simple breathing pattern in the heart centre and Agni centre (between eyebrows). At one point, you'll have glimpses which are a state of thoughtless Mind. It takes time depending on the karmic debts.

There are two types of people; one who would realize and self-motivated based on discussions. And others, who tend to experiment through the pains to understand the pleasure. Whoever you are and whatever you do, Analyze your Mind and its behavioural science to get rid of harmful conditioning. Once you have a little energy conserved based on turning in; then focus your attention on breathing techniques and/or Chakra meditation. These are simple and profound practices which are over thosands of years, formulated by the sages of India.

These steps will transcend and help you lead a noble life; not by means of others imposing it on you, perhaps through your inner revelations. In my view, you should learn from the mistakes and move on. Don't hanker on the past as it has taught you something, just learn from it and move. Your memory would help you realize the sensations of pain and the instances that have caused you with a little research would help you comprehend MIND.

The mind is a tool that God has provided you to use it enjoy in limitations through the senses and transcend to looking at the center using mind, and it's thinking process to get over conditioning. Finally, you will arrive back home. Yoga is the balance in using the senses. You will need to realize by dropping conditioning in mind, by using mind as a vehicle to realize the inner consciousness.

There is none called a saint unless realized to the fullest or perhaps the subconsciousness mind has not surfaced yet. A real Guru is the one who has transcended, the one who is aware of the functioning of mind, body and spirit. There is nobody called a sinner as the society is primarily responsible for the condition of mind as we discussed sixteen sampath causing your characterization. The society should educate about the basics of BODY, MIND and SOUL The energy at the source has been poisoned, and the sexual vital fluid has been exploited in mindless robots.

You have to help yourself by practicing and by living passionately in realizing the inner self, which God has endowed you with! God works in pattern, precision and regularity in all his manifestations; hence, he wouldn't have made a mistake by creating human consciousness with mind. The ultimate challenge is to drop the conditioning!

It depends on how much you are holding on to the shell of conditioning; if you learn to drop like a snake dropping its skin. All your miseries, anguish will disappear. It will melt away with the heart filled in eternal love, the purity of consciousness. The mind aligned with the super consciousness state would yield all secrets of Nature, by expanding the mind to the fullest.

Now, let us analyze the usage of mind in the process of thinking, and contemplation.

Process of Thinking

One of the intrinsic qualities of mind is 'THINKING'. If you think about an Object, the mind becomes it. Perhaps it transforms to the qualities of the subject itself. Just think about an Ocean, Sun and the stars and the eternity. You would feel better, isn't it? The irony is that MIND has the ability to expand by thinking. This is one of the techniques with profound wisdom formulated by Swamiji, a contemporary Siddha of South. India with the expansion of mind through visualization;

In this technique, you will expand the mind by visualization. You'd visualize SUN, and the STARS and the mental frequency reduce gradually. Finally you will end up merging with the cosmic consciousness which is known as the **'Divine Dark Fluid'**. Your mind intercepts peace for a split second. If you can achieve this for an extended period of time, there is a possibility of total realization and Enlightenment!!! These are profound techniques of the Vedic scripts of the ancient Indian school of Yoga system.

One of the ancient sage Vishwamitra had indicated that you can see heaven alive. Perhaps the first sage who had proclaimed heaven exist within the mind. The disciple Thirisangu asks:

Thirisangu: "Maha Muni, can you help me?"

Vishwamitra says: "Of course." You can find heaven while you're alive. He instructs him to expand his mind to visualize the eternal consciousness. This story is very significant as its deft all myth's about the hell and heaven. It is a metaphor of a conditioned mind Vs. the expanded mind. Your expanded state of mind is heaven. When your heart is filled with love, it is heaven! Now, let us try to expand mind to the cosmic consciousness. Just drop all your tension and feel relaxed. Enjoy the eternal tour.

Expanding Mind to Cosmos

A simple exercise to follow. You'll start focusing on chakra centre's, those who're initiated. For rest, it will be focusing on breathing pattern at the prime centres of base of the spine, then heart centre. Finally, between the eyebrows and then transcend using thought by visualizing moon, sun and the stars, planets and galaxies. The Hindu Vedic scriptures revealed mind can assume shape, and it can expand to the infinite. What you think is what you essentially become!!! When you start expanding the mind to the cosmos, you become the truth itself as you have it in the subject at the center of the mind itself.

The technique is so profound that you start visualizing which your inner revelation of Truth. And you start finding your own glimpses of truth if practiced diligently over a period of time.This is based on ancient Indian mystic revelations, which is a unique way of expanding your mind; as mind can take shape, it becomes the object as the subject. You will eventually drop the visualization as there will be no need for it once it becomes your reality.

Anecdote (Three Wise Men)

Once there was a voyage to the Vancouver of Canada. And the three passengers started from North England. A Scientist, Christian Father, and a potter; The Scientist was feeling immensely proud in analyzing various facts and physics, Engineering while he was travelling, while the philosopher was arguing.

Well Gentlemen. I am Jack Hellman. I am a Scientist with a firm handshake, holding the hat to the left. How do you do?

Thanks! I am fine. "My name is Chris Harrington". I am a church – father in North Hampton. Each of them continued, non-stop when the Engines were cranking in the mid-of the sea. The noise of the plates with English omelets and French toast, both of them kept talking while the other poor fellow was agape, listening to the conversation.

Chris: Jack, you gotta learn the life essentials of what the Bible says.

Jack: Thank you father! You know I am a renowned Scientist in town, researching atom and wave Nature.

Chris: Lord is the Father and you are all son of God.

Chris: I gotta analyze it theoretically…

It became an argument in everything as they kept discussing through dinner;

Well. Gentlemen what do you do.

I am a potter, just expert in what I am doing and enjoy swimming.

Pooh! As both of them took off their hats after a long debate.

Poor fellow as they chuckled, while pouring a glass of red-wine. It tastes wonderful, with a bright coat shimmering in the moon light. Both of them continued with the debate non-stop.

After a while, the captain made an announcement…

"'Ladies and Gentlemen' – Emergency. We have a problem and wear the life jacket and jump into Ocean as the ship has hit a major rock, and it will blast at any moment."

"He counted from TEN, NINE….."

Oh my GOD! Both of them exclaimed.

The poor fellow said, 'Do you guys swim?'

I have studied about it, but don't know. Both of them yelled in chorus. And the poor fellow jumped into the sea and asked them to follow him. Which they couldn't.

"Indeed, a real practice make man perfect" instead of talking about philosophy, it's worth experiencing it!

End of Session # 13

Day 12 – Session # 14
Hold on to the Convictions of Truth

Last but not least, I am going to teach you about the convictions of truth based on the Hindu mythology. A few videos to watch. Sit back and relax.

We have discussed Mind, and the lineage to Nature. How can it become your inner revelations, unless you practice methods of analyzing conditioning etc. As we discussed in the earlier chapters.

The fact is that you should hold on to the convictions of truth. As you realize Nature is the '**CAUSE and EFFECT**' system, It is apparent God is descending as results.

As Bhagvat Gita says:

'I'll reveal myself to you as results.'

The above statement indicates the **CAUSE and EFFECT** theory as Nature itself manifesting as results. If you do it incorrectly, confronting the laws of Nature, you'll end up in pains. What happens if you do overeat? You will have to face the consequences of an upset stomach. This is a simple example and no need for any philosophy. You will need to realize the senses by paying attention to the situation. The emerging thoughts, actions, work, sex, and rest etc.

You should counsel yourself; analyze the limited happiness created by these senses, with the limitations of senses. If you need eternal bliss, the only way is to transcend the senses. Enjoyment in moderation, as we discussed in one of the golden Facets of wisdom;

Rule # 7 Hold on to the Convictions of Truth

What is the point in worrying about the results? By the time you're worrying, the past instance is gone. Either way you have to be prepared for a result and it will come as per the Nature's Divine justice. It is the time right now, to analyze your painful sensations, and contemplate and counsel by holding on to centre 'The Truth' itself. This will heal your condition and eleavte to the higher plane of life.

I like a story of 'Bhakta Prahalad', who is son of a demon king, 'Hiranya', who was against Lord Krishna. The child's conviction was to such an extent; the story portrays his convictions of truth.

Let's watch this video. Dr. plays the video!!!

The demon king, his father asks him:

'Son, do not chant the name of Hari. He is our enemy'

Prahalad: Quietly he goes out and sings hymns of Shri Hari... as this:

"Om Namo Narayana
Om Namo Narayana"

I sing, and dance chanting this mantra.

What else can give you salvation and peace?

In life...the only mantra that gives you ultimate pleasure in life!!!

And there is nothing else.

Beyond and above;

He goes to a state of trance by singing!

Narayana...Narayana...Narayana;

Om Namo Narayana....over hundred times and he fall down in the trance state.

The demon King; finally decides to kill his son, ruthlessly by various techniques including an elephant to kill him. And the elephant looks at the eyes of a child who is graciously chanting

185

the mantra, with so much of bliss and his lips chanting: 'OM Namo Narayana' continuously without fearing any consequences, even without fearing death.

It is a significant story of Prahlad, who had surrendered himself totally to the blissful Nature. His conviction of truth was total, and there was no doubt.

Such conviction of truth is rare in the evolution of human consciousness for a child and the demon king calls out for an ultimatum in the courtyard.

Ok. 'Show me your Hari', where the hell is he now?

The child says, he is there everywhere.

'In every simple matter. Here, now, and he is everywhere!!'

He is right here now, listening to you speak!

'Oh, then show me.'

"See...Here, just observe the pillar. He is right there in the pillar,' he pointed out to the large pillar in the palace; the king ordered his soldier to break open the pillar.

The pillar breaks open and there he goes.

Narasimha, a half GOD with an animal face of a Lion appears in front of the Demon King, and he kills him.

Remember, whatever you do through the senses will result in frustrations, unless you understand the limitations of each of the senses. You cannot claim total bliss in these experiences. There is no need to be hankering for the experiences of sex, or happiness in eating as they are extremely momentary and subject to the limitations of senses. Just think how much you can taste food, or how much more you can make love, you will be tired and bored of the futile experiences!

Either you can experiment yourself or comprehend intellectually through the reasoning. Either way you will come to a point in life that nothing seems to be fulfilling, and you will hanker for something eternal. It will be the perfect moment to take a quantum leap into eternal consciousness;

Do not even hanker for eternal and do not hold your Guru or perhaps stay in an ashram forever, if you do. Perhaps that will be futile too. The best way is Zen like; understand, learn from the ashram; and go back to the inner consciousness. Just keep learning, let the conscious grow and fulfil the eternal needs. And no other senses can give you that. If you are intelligent, you will find it real soon. As you grow biologically, how you would be able to comprehend that experiences are limited, unless you perceive things beyond senses.

For example, if you are learning Engineering, you will say that the high school math is much simpler. Unless you are able to expand the mind to the eternal love by opening your heart, how would you comprehend there is ecstasy, bliss. Keep contemplating on these positive emotions, as I have explained earlier, hold on to these experiences, and research your sensations. Your life will be extremely exciting, and bring in your consciousness into everything you do from the smallest of things in every split second. Once you regain the lost touch of the consciousness, the inner light will grow tremendously and accept everything gracefully!!!

The convictions of truth should be your life time endeavour. You should realize the emotions and behaviour that has taken you to where you are right now, just realize and transcend.

Often Zen techniques portray moment to moment awareness in every action, which is indicated in Bhagvat Gita as the 'Karma Yoga' by practicing action in the state of detached attachment in total awareness.

Mr. Martin thanks Dr. Richard for teaching the simple and profound techniques to help in succeed.

Martin, 'Here is the souvenir' as he passes on the beautiful golden palette with the 7 Golden Rules of Zen Wisdom embossed on it.

You've mastered the 7 Golden Rules of Zen Wisdom:

The 7 Golden Rules of Zen Wisdom

1. Identify Your '**SENSATIONS**';

2. Look '**BEYOND**' the Sensations;

3. Enjoyment in '**MODERATION**';

4. Know Your '**CONDITIONING**';

5. Realize '**MIND**' and the lineage to Eternity;

6. PRACTICE '**AWARENESS**' and

7. Hold on to the convictions of '**TRUTH**'

Mr. Martin, 'This is very significant and I've handed over the golden palette which will help the younger generation and many more generations to come. Go to the World and teach them about the '7 Golden Rules of Zen Wisdom '. It took me more than couple of decades to master it based on my research in Western Psychiatry, and the Eastern philosophy including Zen Wisdom.

I am sure this research will help the younger generations to contemplate and succeed in their endeavor. Go teach them all to transcend addictions and help them explore the frontiers of mind beyond mundane pleasures.

Good Luck my Friend! Dr. Richard awards him a souvenir, a beautiful '7 Golden Rules of Zen Wisdom' Golden palette along with a handwritten letter.

End of Session # 14

Mr. Martin's memory flashes back to the presence with the flashing cameras on stage.

Martin continues…

"Today, I am here because of this gentleman named Dr. Richard, who is not here today to see me succeed in my endeavour. The man who showed me virtues in life by teaching the subtle techniques of '7 Golden Rules of Zen Wisdom."

He shows the Golden palette to everyone in the crowd. "The Seven Golden Rules of Zen Wisdom."

'Today, I am standing in front of you all with confidence after achieving success in my life.'

I am honoured to indicate that I was one among the student of Dr. Richard, who has helped me in realizing the conditioning. From that day, I trasnformed from the mundane plane of life to the state of awareness. Today. It's his philosophy which is enlightening millions of students, and adults those who are brave enough to venture into the inner frontiers of mind.

"Today, I am deeply sadened to miss my teacher, my friend, philosopher and a guide who has helped me reach here to this stage."

And he pauses for a while, may the soul rest in peace.

"I couldn't have even moved an inch in my life without his guidance, transforming my drunken life to the Divine life of wisdom."

'Indeed, I am blessed to have a teacher like Dr. Richard. I salute his services to the World. The last letter from Dr. indicated these words that I cannot forget in my life time.'

He showcases the letter to the audience, a handwritten letter from Dr. Richard:

2005 – South Carolina.

Dear Martin,

You're unique if you remember this. I have taught you the "7 Golden Rules of Zen Wisdom" and you've grasped it very well. Practise it and teach the World. Indeed, World is one and help the younger generations to succeed in life by getting over addictions. It is your responsibility to teach every student to realize the inner values to gain strength and wisdom.

Good Luck!

This letter is my motivation, and my responsibility. It is your motivation and responsibility to practise. I read this every morning!

I thank you each of you for the honour. I'll not stop teaching the '**7 Golden Rules of Zen Wisdom**' until my last breadth.

Thank you Ladies and Gentlemen!!!

●●

Epilogue

The revelation of truth is your birth right, and there is

no need to follow a belief based system. You have the ability to realize truth, based on the past sequence of events so far. The mind is capable of expanding beyond the frontiers and transcend addictions if you believe you could achieve. You have the ability to realize the inner consciousness, using mind as a tool to expand to the eternity by following the techniques discussed.

The duality in mind can be analyzed, and conditioning can be uprooted through the constant spiritual practices that were discussed in the '7 Golden Rules of Zen Wisdom; All you have to do is to unleash the energy towards analysis by means of self-enquiry, practices and eliminate the conditioning of the past and the reactive behaviour. The harmful behaviour should be replaced by inquisitive reasoning. The behavioural science helps us analyze facts of human consciousness, behaviour and its extension as Mind.

The thoughts are the roots of sensations, and the Mind is a wave which dissolves into feelings, emotions. The ultimate consciousness is the centre of mind which perceives it through the senses as pleasure or pain or peace. This is the ultimate science, and there is no need for any medications. There is nowhere to go, and nobody to ask for help, rather your inner consciousness is the saviour.

There is a saying practice makes a man perfect'; without practice and a plan of action you cannot succeed in any endeavour. You should treat each of the conditioning at the grass root levels, and allow the conscious mind be engrossed in alignment with the Divine Nature.

The emotional bubble in the subconscious mind will emerge as you grow biologically, as well as spiritually. The bubble will try to break into the conscious mind as emotions, thus creating chaos. You have to be diligently practicing virtues, based on the realization and revelations of truth to achieve success in every stage of life.

The culmination of the East and the West is the final climax in the evolution of super consciousness. The Sixth sense will be crowned, as the newer community has just begun transcending Karl Marx's socialism to the Spiritualism; The Spiritualism with Science will be leading in all aspects of teaching Religiousness, ways of living by teaching meditation and behavioural analysis to support each other in the endeavour of consciousness.

You're the master as you've mastered the '**7 Golden Rules of Zen Wisdom**'.

●●